NCLEX-PN®
FLASHCARDS

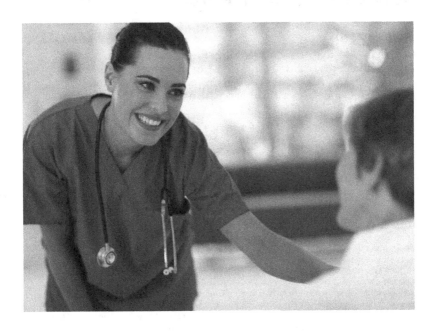

Rebekah Warner, RN, BSN

Research & Education Association
Visit our website at: www.rea.com

Research & Education Association
61 Ethel Road West
Piscataway, New Jersey 08854
E-mail: info@rea.com

NCLEX-PN® Flashcard Book

Published 2017

Copyright © 2015 by Research & Education Association, Inc.
Prior editions copyright © 2009, 2008 by Research & Education
Association, Inc. All rights reserved. No part of this book may be
reproduced in any form without permission of the publisher.

Printed in the United States of America

ISBN-13: 978-0-7386-1178-5
ISBN-10: 0-7386-1178-6

Cover image © Catherine Yeulet/iStock/Thinkstock

REA® is a registered trademark of
Research & Education Association, Inc.

Welcome to REA's NCLEX-PN Flashcard Book

If you have completed your nursing school studies and are getting ready to take the National Council Licensure Examination for Practical Nurses (NCLEX-PN), our *NCLEX-PN Flashcard Book* will help you prepare.

Written by a critical care nurse with years of practical experience, our 425 must-study questions cover the four major Client Needs categories and six subcategories tested on the NCLEX-PN exam:

- Safe and Effective Care Environment
  - Coordinated Care
  - Safety and Infection Control
- Health Promotion and Maintenance
- Psychosocial Integrity
- Physiological Integrity
  - Basic Care and Comfort
  - Pharmacological Therapies
  - Reduction of Risk Potential
  - Physiological Adaptation

Each flashcard is labeled with the corresponding NCLEX-PN test category, so you can target the topics where you need the most review. Refer to our handy index for fast access to the full range of topics covered.

When you've mastered the material in this book, you'll be well equipped to pass the NCLEX-PN exam and on your way to a rewarding nursing career.

Good luck on the test!

About REA

Founded in 1959, Research & Education Association (REA) is dedicated to publishing the finest and most effective educational materials—including study guides and test preps—for students of all ages. Today, REA's wide-ranging catalog is a leading resource for students, teachers, and other professionals. Visit *www.rea.com* to see a complete listing of all our titles.

Acknowledgments

We would like to thank Larry B. Kling, Vice President, Editorial, for his overall direction; Pam Weston, Publisher, for setting the quality standards for production integrity and managing the publication to completion; Kelli Wilkins, Editor, for project management; Claudia Petrilli, Graphic Designer, for designing our cover; Ellen Gong for proofreading; and TCS for typesetting the manuscript.

About Our Author

Rebekah Warner, **RN**, is an expert in critical care nursing. She received her BSN degree from Roberts Wesleyan College in 2004. While in nursing school, Rebekah was inducted into the Sigma Theta Tau International Honor Society of Nursing. Her certifications include Basic Life Support (BLS), Advanced Cardiac Life Support (ACLS), and Cardio-Pulmonary Resuscitation (CPR).

Safe and Effective Care Environment:
Coordinated Care

Q–1

The LPN/LVN is aware that state boards of nursing share what common components? Select all that apply.

(A) Establish requirements for entry into practice for RNs and LPNs.
(B) Determine each state's pay scale for licensed nurses.
(C) Oversee the discipline for all licensed healthcare workers in each state.
(D) Define the scope of practice for RNs and LPN/LVNs.
(E) Identify legal titles for nurses.

Physiological Integrity:
Basic Care and Comfort

Q–2

The LPN/LVN observes a nursing assistant applying a client's antiembolism stockings. What is the appropriate routine for these stockings?

(A) The nursing assistant is applying the stockings just after assisting the patient with ROM leg exercises.
(B) The nursing assistant is applying the stockings just before assisting the patient out of bed in the morning.
(C) The nursing assistant is applying the stockings at night as the patient is getting ready to go to sleep.
(D) The nursing assistant is applying the stockings after observing the color and temperature of the skin.

Answers

A–1

(A), **(D)**, and **(E)** Although each state has its own nurse practice act, they all share the following common components: define the scope of practice; establish requirements for licensure and entry into practice; create a board of nursing to oversee nursing practice; identify legal titles for nurses, such as registered nurse and licensed practical or licensed vocational nurse; define the role and oversight of unlicensed assistive personnel (UAP); and determine what constitutes grounds for disciplinary action for nurses. State boards of nursing would not oversee discipline for all healthcare workers (such as MDs) and would not commonly set the pay scale for nurses.

A–2

(B) The correct and best time for application of antiembolism stockings is in the morning, before the client gets out of bed or after the legs have been elevated for an amount of time. The client's lower extremities should be in a non-dependent position during application to prevent trapping venous blood. Antiembolism stockings are usually worn continuously and should only be removed for the nurse to assess the skin.

Q–3

Mr. Stone is a 32-year-old who recently underwent ORIF (open reduction, internal fixation) surgery for a fractured femur. Over the past few hours the client has started to call the nurse frequently. Mr. Stone has also become more irritable and restless. The best nursing response to this behavior would be:

(A) Encourage the patient to use relaxation techniques to aid with pain management.
(B) Notify the doctor of the patient's behavior.
(C) Ask the patient if there is something on his mind that he'd like to talk about.
(D) Check on and interact with the client frequently until he is calm, and then increase the intervals as he starts to develop trust in the staff.

A–3

(B) Subtle personality changes, restlessness, irritability, or confusion in a patient who has recently sustained a fracture are indications of possible fat emboli that have migrated to the lungs. The physician should be immediately notified of any of these changes to allow for further and immediate testing and evaluation. Encouraging relaxation, therapeutic communication, and methods to improve trust are interventions that do not deal with the dangerous condition that the symptoms suggest.

Physiological Integrity:
Physiological Adaptation

Q-4

Mr. Godfry, a warehouse worker, presented to the Emergency Department with an acute onset of severe lower back pain, muscle spasms, and radiation of pain into the buttocks and leg. The physician suspects that Mr. Godfry has a herniated lumbar intervertebral disk. During assessment, the nurse asks Mr. Godfry to describe the characteristics of the pain. Which of the following is an aggravating factor of the condition suspected by the physician?

(A) Sneezing
(B) Chewing
(C) Talking
(D) Bed rest

Physiological Integrity:
Basic Care and Comfort

Q-5

The LPN/LVN is assessing a client's halo traction to ensure it is applied appropriately. Which of the following observations indicates proper use of this device?

(A) The client states his pain is "bearable."
(B) The client is able to wiggle his toes comfortably.
(C) The client is not able to turn his head from side to side.
(D) There is a finger-width of space between the client's skin and the traction device.

A-4

(A) Pain associated with a herniated intervertebral disk is aggravated by actions that increase intraspinal pressure, such as bending, lifting, or straining. Sneezing or coughing involves an amount of straining. The movement associated with chewing and talking does not usually affect this condition. Although bed rest can aggravate symptoms of other conditions, it is usually a relieving factor for herniated disk pain.

A-5

(C) Halo traction is used to keep the neck neutrally aligned and immobilized. The best confirmation that the halo traction is applied properly is that the client is unable to turn his head from side to side. Traction does not control pain. The patient should be medicated for pain as appropriate. Traction fits each person differently. Although it should fit in a way that avoids compromising the patient's skin integrity, there is no rule for the distance between the device and the skin or body part.

Physiological Integrity:
Reduction of Risk Potential

Q–6

Mrs. Fischner, a 55-year-old client, presents to her physician that she has stiffness and pain in her joints that "never seems to go away." After laboratory tests, the physician diagnoses rheumatoid arthritis. The results of which laboratory test most likely led to the physician's diagnosis?

(A) Serum creatinine
(B) Erythrocyte sedimentation rate (ESR)
(C) International normalized ratio (INR)
(D) Fasting lipid panel

Physiological Integrity:
Physiological Adaptation

Q–7

Mrs. Fischner's physician diagnosed that she has rheumatoid arthritis. With this condition, the client's chief complaint is persistent joint pain and stiffness. Pain and stiffness associated with rheumatoid arthritis is most often first noticed in the joints of which of the following?

(A) Hands
(B) Arms
(C) Legs
(D) Neck

A–6

(B) Erythrocyte sedimentation rate (ESR) is the best diagnostic indicator of rheumatoid arthritis. ESR is a nonspecific test that indicates the presence of an inflammatory disease when elevated. Rheumatoid arthritis is one of a number of disease processes that will elevate this serum level. Serum creatinine is used to evaluate kidney function. International normalized ratio (INR) tests the effectiveness of anticoagulation therapy, usually with the drug Warfarin (Coumadin). A fasting lipid panel measures the cholesterol and lipid levels and ratios that are present in the blood when the levels are not affected by recent food ingestion.

A–7

(A) Clients with rheumatoid arthritis usually experience discomfort in the proximal finger joints of the hands before any other joints of the body. Although rheumatoid arthritis can eventually spread to any or every joint, the symptoms of rheumatoid arthritis usually are noticed in the finger and hand joints prior to the joints of the arms, legs, and neck.

Safe and Effective Care Environment:
Coordinated Care

Q–8

A client has spent the last half hour screaming loudly and cursing anyone who comes in his room. The nurse enters the room and grabs the client's foot and yells, "Be quiet. I have heard all I want to hear from you tonight." What legal act could this nurse be charged with?

(A) Assault
(B) Battery
(C) Defamation
(D) Invasion of privacy

Physiological Integrity:
Reduction of Risk Potential

Q–9

Mrs. Jones, a 60-year-old client with advanced diabetic neuropathy is two days post-op from a right-above-the-knee amputation. During assessment, the LPN/LVN asks the client if she is experiencing any pain. Mrs. Jones replies, "I've been afraid to mention it. I know my right foot isn't there anymore, but I feel it aching." Which of the following is the most accurate explanation for this sensation?

(A) "You may feel pain in the tissues near the incision site, which is known as referred pain."
(B) "You may be experiencing a psychosomatic pain response as a result of the loss you are experiencing."
(C) "You may be experiencing intractable pain, which can be controlled well with the appropriate narcotics."
(D) "You may be experiencing a sensation called 'phantom pain' from the site of the amputation."

A–8

(B) Battery is physical contact with another person without that person's consent. This contact can include touching a person's body, clothing, chair, or bed. A charge of battery can be made even if the contact did not cause physical harm to the individual. A charge of assault is an act that involves a threat or attempt to do bodily harm. Defamation is an act that harms a person's reputation and good name. Invasion of privacy means that person has the right to expect that the individual and property will be left alone. The nurse grabbed the client's foot, which constitutes battery.

A–9

(D) Phantom pain is a real sensation that some people feel after loss of a limb or other body part. This can be felt differently by different individuals. Many have described it as burning, cramping, or itching. Some people sense that the limb is still there. Referred pain is the sensation of pain localized in an area distant from the actual injury or area of pathology. Psychosomatic pain or illness is a discomfort or array of symptoms caused by mental processes or emotional responses as opposed to physiological causes. Intractable pain is an often unexplainable, severe, and unrelenting pain. Combined therapies are usually necessary to treat intractable pain.

Physiological Integrity:
Basic Care and Comfort

Q–10

Mrs. Jones is in her second post-op day with a right-above-the-knee amputation. She asks the nurse why her stump must be rewrapped every day with an elastic bandage. Which of the following is the most accurate reason for this procedure?

(A) "The bandage absorbs drainage and blood from the incision site."

(B) "The bandage helps shape the stump and shrinks the stump size."

(C) "The bandage prevents dehiscence of the incision caused by movement."

(D) "The bandage helps increase circulation to the incision site."

Physiological Integrity:
Reduction of Risk Potential

Q–11

A client has just returned to the hospital room from a liver biopsy. Which of the following is a complication that the LPN/LVN should be aware could occur within the first few hours following this procedure?

(A) Hemorrhage

(B) Infection

(C) Tension pneumothorax

(D) Anaphylaxis

A–10

(B) The site of a new amputation will develop a large amount of edema. Stump wrapping with an elastic bandage shrinks and shapes the stump for prosthesis construction. Therefore, answer (B) is correct. The prosthesis will not be sized and constructed until the stump is cone shaped and the size is no longer changing. Gauze bandages are used to absorb blood and drainage. Dehiscence is the separation of the edges or reopening of a closed incision. With appropriate suturing, normal movement should not cause dehiscence. Antiembolism stockings are used to aid circulation in uncompromised limbs.

A–11

(A) The most common complication following a liver biopsy is bleeding, which can lead to severe hemorrhage. This is because of the vascular nature of the liver and the possibility for escape of blood through the needle insertion site. The correct answer is option (A). Infection could occur at the puncture site, but this complication occurs gradually, not within a few hours. A tension pneumothorax occurs when air enters the pleural cavity and becomes trapped after the lung has been punctured or lacerated. This would induce immediate symptoms during the biopsy and would not develop over the hours following the procedure. Anaphylaxis is a severe allergic response. This should not occur with a liver biopsy.

Q–12

Mrs. Jamison has just returned from a biopsy of her liver. Which of the following instructions provided by the nurse is inaccurate for care following this procedure?

(A) The nurse tells the client to "avoid coughing or straining for the next few hours, if possible."

(B) The nurse instructs the client to "inhale and exhale deeply several times and then exhale and hold your breath at the end of expiration." The client is instructed to repeat this activity every 10 minutes for the first couple of hours after the procedure.

(C) The nurse instructs the client to lie "on [her] right side with a pillow under [her] rib cage."

(D) The nurse states that the client will have to "avoid heavy lifting and any strenuous activity for one week" following the procedure.

Answers

A–12

(B) This answer refers to the instructions the nurse would give to a client during the liver biopsy procedure. Holding the breath immobilizes the diaphragm and chest wall to avoid perforation of the diaphragm during insertion of the biopsy needle. Following a liver biopsy, coughing or straining could lead to straining of the puncture site and escape of blood. Lying on the right side compresses the puncture site against the chest wall to impede bleeding at the site, and leaning on a pillow will provide comfort in this position for a longer time period. Cautious activity reduces the risk for blood escaping from the biopsy puncture site.

Q-13

The LPN/LVN is providing blood pressure readings at a local convenience store for members of the community. For which of the following client readings should the nurse recommend follow-up with the client's primary doctor within a period of two months?

(A) $\dfrac{114}{78}$

(B) $\dfrac{120}{82}$

(C) $\dfrac{134}{97}$

(D) $\dfrac{138}{89}$

Answers

(C) Normal blood pressure readings range between 100 to 140 systolic and 60 to 90 diastolic. The Joint National Committee on Detection, Evaluation, and Treatment of High Blood Pressure (2003) recommends that if either a systolic reading between 140 and 149 or a diastolic reading of 90 to 99 is obtained, the client's blood pressure should be rechecked in 2 months following the initial reading. The correct answer is (C). In this answer the diastolic reading is above normal range. All other answers are within normal blood pressure range.

Safe and Effective Care Environment:
Safety and Infection Control

Q–14

The LPN/LVN caring for Mr. Braxton, a 69-year-old client admitted to the extended stay facility, notices that he has an unsteady gait. Select each of the following that are appropriate nursing actions for the LPN/LVN in this situation (choose all answer choices that apply):

(A) Ensure the client's room is free of clutter or obstacles.
(B) Provide adequate lighting to the client's room.
(C) Make sure the call light stays on the nightstand at all times.
(D) Place throw rugs around the client's room.
(E) Have the client sit in a chair with a vest restraint applied.
(F) Keep the client's bed in its lowest position with all four side rails up.

Physiological Integrity:
Basic Care and Comfort

Q–15

During routine vital signs, the LPN/LVN auscultates a BP of $\frac{180}{98}$. How long should the LPN/LVN wait before inflating the cuff to recheck this reading?

(A) 15 seconds
(B) 30 seconds
(C) 1 minute
(D) 2 minutes

Answers

A–14

(A) and (B) are the only correct answers to this question. Removing obstacles and clutter from the client's room decreases the risk that the client will trip over an item. Adequate lighting ensures the client can see appropriately when moving around the room. It may not be appropriate for the call light to be on the nightstand if it is not within the client's reach. The client should be able to reach the call light at all times. Throw rugs are not permanently fixed to the floor surface and are therefore fall hazards. Keeping the bed in its lowest position is appropriate, but keeping all of the side rails up increases the distance a client could fall when trying to get out of bed.

A–15

(D) The American Heart Association (AHA) recommends waiting two minutes before repeating a blood pressure reading at the same site. This is to decrease venous congestion. The correct answer is (D). All of the other answers give too short of a time span between cuff inflations.

Q–16

The LPN/LVN walks into a client's room and observes that the client immediately begins to display grand mal seizure activity. Select all of the following nursing actions that should be performed at this time:

(A) Turn the client onto her side with her neck flexed.
(B) Apply soft wrist restraints for the duration of the seizure.
(C) Maintain an airway by inserting a tongue depressor into the client's mouth.
(D) Trigger the facility's procedure for emergency response.
(E) Raise the side rails.
(F) Remove any loose items from the client's bed.

Q–17

Mrs. Palmer, a client with Parkinson's disease, is admitted to an extended-stay nursing facility. Up until this point she has been living on her own. Which of the following assessments is most significant in developing the plan of care?

(A) Mrs. Palmer states she dislikes beef but will eat it once in a while if it is cooked well.
(B) Mrs. Palmer talks frequently about how much she misses living on her own.
(C) Mrs. Palmer has a difficult time eating at dinner due to tremors.
(D) Mrs. Palmer states her only living relative is her daughter who lives across the state and seldom visits.

A–16

(A), **(D)**, **(E)**, and **(F)** should all be selected. Client safety is the top priority during a convulsion. Important actions to maintain safety include placing the client in a side-lying position to allow drainage of oral secretions, activating emergency response, removing all items from the bed that could cause bodily harm, and raising and padding the side rails. During a seizure a client will be experiencing strong spasms that cause muscle contractions. Restraining a client could cause injury to the musculoskeletal system. Muscle contractions in the jaw cause the client's teeth to clench. Never attempt to insert anything into clenched teeth. Doing so may cause injury to the teeth and lips.

A–17

(C) Although it is important to consider all client needs holistically, the highest concern in establishing a plan of care is the physiological needs of the client. Physiological needs include all ADLs (activities of daily living). ADLs are basic needs, such as eating, moving, dressing, toileting, and other personal hygiene. Answer (C) is the correct answer because it is the only assessment that indicates a physical hindrance to a physiological need.

Safe and Effective Care Environment:
Coordinated Care

Q–18

Which of the following is a correct initial nursing action to be performed by the LPN/LVN when a client with a physician-written DNR order goes into cardiac arrest?

(A) Notify the physician.
(B) Initiate the emergency response system.
(C) Perform rescue breathing and chest compressions.
(D) Move the crash cart into the room beside the client's bed.

Safe and Effective Care Environment:
Coordinated Care

Q–19

The nurse is caring for a client who has a habit of making very inappropriate statements to any caregiver. What must the nurse do to decrease the risk of this client accusing the nurse of defamation of character? Select all that apply.

(A) Only speak negatively about the client to other healthcare professionals.
(B) Refrain from mentioning any client in a public area such as the cafeteria.
(C) Ensure that the nurse is never alone with the client.
(D) Limit documentation of the client's actions to the actual words the client speaks.
(E) Confront the client about the inappropriate speech so that others can hear the interaction.

Answers

(A) A DNR or "Do Not Resuscitate" order indicates that in the case of cardiac or respiratory arrest, no lifesaving treatment will be initiated. In order for DNR procedures to stand, a written physician's order must be documented in the medical record. Initiating the emergency response system is not necessary for a client with a DNR order. Emergency actions, such as rescue breathing and chest compressions, will not be performed. A crash cart containing emergency medications and a defibrillator will not be used on this client. The physician should be notified of the client's status. Answer (A) is correct.

(B) and **(D)** Nurses are at risk for defamation of character suits if they make negative comments in public areas (elevators, cafeterias) or assert opinions regarding a client's character in the medical record. The nurse should refrain from negative speech about any client. The only remarks between healthcare professionals should concern the information needed for care of the client. Defamation of character concerns the nurse's speech that others can hear so the nurse should not confront the client about the client's speech where others can hear. Ensuring that the nurse is never alone with the client would not prevent the client from filing a defamation of character suit.

Safe and Effective Care Environment:
Coordinated Care

Q–20

Mrs. Strobell is walking in the hallway with the nursing assistant. She experiences sudden onset of angina. Which of the following should be the first action taken by the LPN/LVN?

(A) Call the physician immediately.
(B) Instruct Mrs. Strobell to relax and discontinue all muscle movement.
(C) Tell the nursing assistant to help Mrs. Strobell walk back to her bed slowly and lie down.
(D) Retrieve a wheelchair and an oxygen tank from the supply room and transport Mrs. Strobell back to her room.

Physiological Integrity:
Reduction of Risk Potential

Q–21

Mrs. Garner is visiting her obstetrician at 12-weeks gestation. Which of the following laboratory findings would indicate the need for intervention in the client's prenatal care?

(A) Serum glucose of 96 g/dL
(B) White blood cell count of 13 mm³
(C) Hematocrit of 30%
(D) Hemoglobin of 12 g/dL

Answers

(B) Angina is pain in the chest that is caused by an insufficient flow of oxygen to the cardiac muscle. Muscle activity that occurs with movement increases the oxygen demand of the cardiac muscle. Discontinuing all movement will decrease the oxygen demand of the muscle. It is important to administer supplemental oxygen as soon as possible, and the client should not walk or stand any more than necessary while experiencing angina. While a wheelchair and an oxygen tank are being retrieved, the nurse can instruct the client to remain still and relax as much as possible. Of the answer choices, answer (B) is the correct initial action. Once back in her room, Mrs. Strobell can be assisted to bed to lie down.

(C) In pregnancy, a client's hematocrit should be between 32% and 46%. A hematocrit of 30% indicates slight anemia. Normal serum glucose in pregnancy is 65 to 110 g/dL. Normal white blood cell count in pregnancy is 9 to 15 mm^3. Normal hemoglobin in pregnancy is 11 to 13 g/dL.

Safe and Effective Care Environment:
Safety and Infection Control

Q–22

Which of the following should be initiated for a client suspected of having meningitis?

(A) Standard precautions
(B) Contact precautions
(C) Droplet precautions
(D) Airborne precautions

Physiological Integrity:
Physiological Adaptation

Q–23

Which of the following assessments is the most important when examining a client who is suspected to be experiencing a CVA (cerebrovascular accident)?

(A) Vital signs
(B) Motor response
(C) Integrity of the airway
(D) Level of consciousness (LOC)

Answers

A–22

(C) The correct answer is droplet precautions. Most forms of meningitis are transmitted from the secretion droplets of those who are infected. Standard precautions are used with all clients, whether or not they are known or thought to be infected with a transmittable disease. Airborne and contact precautions would not be effective in preventing transmission of this pathogen.

A–23

(D) The first thing to assess in a client who displays signs and symptoms of a CVA (cerebrovascular accident) is level of consciousness (LOC). LOC most quickly and accurately indicates the level of brain function. This is also the first assessment in the ABCs of emergency response procedures. Airway integrity would be assessed after unconsciousness is confirmed. If the client is conscious, vital signs and motor response should then be assessed. Vital sign changes and motor response deficits give further information about the characteristics of the CVA.

Physiological Integrity:
Reduction of Risk Potential

Q–24

The LPN/LVN is caring for a one-day-old male neonate. After feeding the infant 0.5 oz of formula, he is burped and placed in the crib. Which of the following is the ideal position for the LPN/LVN to lay the infant?

(A) Right lateral with the crib mattress flat
(B) Right lateral with the foot of the crib mattress elevated
(C) Left lateral with the foot of the crib mattress elevated
(D) Prone with the head of the crib mattress elevated

Physiological Integrity:
Pharmacological Therapies

Q–25

The physician writes an order for a client to receive Digoxin 0.08 mg IV q day. The mixture of Digoxin in the vial contains 0.05 mg of medication in 1 mL of solution. The nurse preparing the medication should draw up how much of the solution?

Answers

A–24

(A) The right lateral position promotes gastric emptying and emptying of the oropharynx. Therefore, answer (A) is the best answer. Elevating the foot of the crib mattress would increase the risk of aspiration. The prone position is almost always discouraged for an infant due to research that has connected this position with SIDS (sudden infant death syndrome).

A–25

ANSWER: 1.6 mL
RATIONALE: Solve for x mL using the following ratio method

$$\frac{0.05 \text{ mg}}{1 \text{ mL}} = \frac{0.08 \text{ mg}}{x \text{ mL}}$$

$$0.05x = 0.08$$

$$x = \frac{0.08}{0.05}$$

$$x = 1.6 \text{ mL solution}$$

Physiological Integrity:
Pharmacological Therapies

Q–26

The LPN/LVN administers the prescribed dose of NPH insulin to a client at 0700. At what time should the peak effects of this medication be expected to take place?

(A) 1700 (5 PM)
(B) 2100 (9 PM)
(C) 1400 (2 PM)
(D) 1100 (11 AM)

Physiological Integrity:
Reduction of Risk Potential

Q–27

The LPN/LVN is preparing to insert a nasogastric tube into the client's gastrointestinal tract. Prior to insertion, the nurse would determine how far to insert the tube by marking the place on the tube that is equal to which of the following distances?

(A) The distance from the tip of the nose to the belly button.
(B) The distance from the top of the head to the top of the ear, to the belly button.
(C) The distance from the tip of the earlobe to the belly button.
(D) The distance from the nose to the earlobe plus the earlobe to the sternum.

Answers

(A) NPH is an intermediate-acting insulin that peaks between 8 and 12 hours after administration. The peak effects of NPH insulin administered at this time would occur between 1500 (3 pm) and 1900 (7 pm). Answer (B) is too late for the peak action of this medication to occur. Answers (C) and (D) are too early for the peak action of this medication to occur.

(D) The length of the nasogastric tubing necessary for each individual client is measured by using the tube to mark off the distance from the tip of the client's nose to the tip of the earlobe and then from the tip of the earlobe to the tip of the sternum. This is approximately the distance from the nares to the stomach, which varies from client to client. The distances of the other answers would not provide an accurate measurement for the desired length.

Physiological Integrity:
Reduction of Risk Potential

Q–28

The distance has been determined and marked on the tubing for inserting a nasogastric tube into a client's gastrointestinal tract. Using all answers provided, arrange the following answer choices into the order of steps that would be followed during insertion of a nasogastric tube:

(A) Lubricate the tip of the NG tube.
(B) Wash hands and put on gloves.
(C) Ask the client to tilt the head forward.
(D) Check tube placement.
(E) Ask the client to hyperextend the neck.
(F) Have the client swallow sips of water while advancing the tube 5 to 10 centimeters with each swallow.

Physiological Integrity:
Physiological Adaptation

Q–29

Which of the following would provide the best information as to whether hemodialysis (HD) has been effective therapy for a client with renal failure?

(A) Checking the client's weight
(B) Measuring intake and output
(C) Checking the potassium level of the client's blood
(D) Monitoring a client's tolerance to exercise

Answers

(B), (A), (E), (C), (F), (D). Prior to any procedure, the nurse should perform appropriate hand-washing procedures and put on gloves. A lubricant is applied to the tubing prior to insertion to ease movement through the gastrointestinal tract. During initial insertion of the tube, the client should hyperextend the neck to reduce the curvature of the nasopharyngeal junction. Once the tube is past the nasopharyngeal junction, the client should tilt the head forward to prevent the tube from going into the larynx. Once in the esophagus, having the client take sips of water while advancing the tube will make the process more natural and prevent discomfort. Once the desired length of the tube is inserted, it is important to confirm that the tube is placed in the stomach and not the lungs.

(A) Hemodialysis (HD) is indicated for clients with fluid volume excess and electrolyte imbalances. Fluid loss or gain is assessed by checking the client's weight at least once a day as well as before and after HD sessions. The amount of weight loss or gain at these times is used to monitor effectiveness of or further need for HD. Measuring intake and output is important to ensure limited fluid intake for clients with renal failure, but this will not indicate HD effectiveness. Clients with renal failure often experience fatigue with exercise, but factors other than those associated with renal failure could cause fatigue. HD is used to regulate serum electrolyte levels (i.e., potassium), but these levels will not indicate overall effectiveness of HD.

Q–30

Which of the following pressure points is most likely to be at risk for developing a pressure wound while a client is in the prone position?

(A) Occiput
(B) Elbows
(C) Toes
(D) Coccyx

Q–31

A 49-year-old male client is admitted to the unit for alcohol withdrawal. The client insists that he had his last drink 4 hours prior. Which of the following medications would the LPN/LVN expect to administer to the client?

(A) Naloxone hydrochloride (Narcan)
(B) Chlordiazepoxide hydrochloride (Librium)
(C) Disulfiram (Antabuse)
(D) Chlorpromazine (Thorazine)

Answers

(**C**) Prone position involves the client lying with the anterior surface of the body compressed against the bed or lying area. The occiput, elbow, and coccyx (also called the tailbone) are all pressure points that would be compromised if the client were to lay with the posterior surface against the bed or lying area. The toes would be compressed against the lying area with the client in the prone position. Therefore, the correct answer is (C).

(**B**) Chlordiazepoxide hydrochloride (Librium) is an antianxiety agent that is used in the treatment of alcohol withdrawal. Naloxone hydrochloride (Narcan) is an antidote for opioids. Narcan is used to reverse the effects of opioid overdose. Disulfiram (Antabuse) is an alcohol deterrent used to treat alcoholism. Antabuse cannot be taken if the client has ingested alcohol in the past 12 hours. Among other uses, chlorpromazine (Thorazine) is most often used to treat psychosis or control nausea and vomiting.

Physiological Integrity:
Pharmacological Therapies

Q–32

Eighty-year-old Mr. Lewis visits the physician at the clinic for his routine check-up. Following the doctor's orders, Mr. Lewis has been taking Amphogel for the past two weeks. Which of the following side effects should the LPN/LVN assess for?

(A) Constipation
(B) Diarrhea
(C) Dizziness
(D) Pruritis

Physiological Integrity:
Pharmacological Therapies

Q–33

Which of the following are appropriate steps that are involved in irrigating a client's eye?

(A) Have the client tilt his/her head toward the opposite eye.
(B) Wash hands and put on gloves.
(C) Irrigate with the solution until the eye is no longer reddened.
(D) Place the drops of solution into the center of the eye.
(E) Place the drops of solution into the inner corner of the eye.
(F) Offer a tissue to the client.

A–32

(A) Aluminum hydroxide (Amphogel) is used for the treatment of ulcers by neutralizing gastric acid. A frequent side effect of this medication is constipation, answer (A). It is uncommon for clients to experience diarrhea, dizziness, or pruritis (itching) from the use of Amphogel.

A–33

(B), (E), and (F) are all correct. Standard precautions, such as hand washing and applying gloves are used any time a health-care worker will come in contact with a patient, especially when handling body orifices or fluids going into or secreted from a patient. The solution should be dropped into the conjunctival sac at the inner canthus (inside corner of the eye). Applying the solution directly to the center of the eye could damage the cornea. A tissue is offered for the client to absorb solution that flows out of the eye. The client should be instructed to tilt his/her head toward the eye being irrigated. The chemical composition of the solution will cause the eye to redden, as would any foreign object that is introduced to the eye.

Safe and Effective Care Environment:
Coordinated Care

Q–34

The LPN/LVN is caring for a client who has just received preoperative sedation. As the LPN/LVN begins to raise the side rail, prior to leaving the room, the client states, "Don't put that up. It makes me feel like a prisoner." After explaining the reason for the raised side rail, the client continues to emphatically refuse to have it raised. What are the LPN/LVN's best actions in caring for this client? Select all that apply.

(A) Raise the side rail and leave the room.
(B) Document the client's refusal to follow standard safety procedures.
(C) Remain in the room with the client until surgery begins.
(D) Notify the registered nurse assigned to the client about the situation.
(E) Contact the surgeon about the client's refusal to have the side rail raised.

Physiological Integrity:
Physiological Adaptation

Q–35

Of the following symptoms, which would indicate that a client has a deficiency of riboflavin?

(A) Ecchymosis
(B) Dry, cracked lips and mouth
(C) Night blindness
(D) Anorexia, weight loss, and fatigue

Answers

(B) and **(D)** If a client is forewarned of a potential hazard and chooses to ignore the warning, the court may hold the client responsible (if the client files suit related to an injury that occurred when the side rails were down). It is essential that the nurse document that the client was warned and that the client disregarded the warning. The nurse does not have the authority to raise the side rails without the client's permission because it would be considered a form of restraint. It is not feasible for the nurse to remain in the client's room waiting for surgery to begin and it would not be appropriate to notify the surgeon of the client's refusal to have the side rails raised. The LPN/LVN would notify the registered nurse.

(B) Insufficient amounts of Riboflavin (or Vitamin B_2) leads to development of dry skin lesions, usually found in or around the mouth. Riboflavin is not stored in the body, and therefore must be restored through dietary supply. Foods that contain riboflavin include dairy products, eggs, whole-grain enriched breads and cereals, liver, and green leafy vegetables. Ecchymosis (bruising) is a result of a decrease in essential clotting factors in the blood, as in Vitamin K deficiency. Night blindness is a result of Vitamin A deficiency. Anorexia, weight loss, and fatigue are symptoms of Thiamin (or Vitamin B_1) deficiency.

Health Promotion and Maintenance

Q–36

During hospitalization, Mrs. Granger is diagnosed with peptic ulcer disease (PUD). The physician has ordered her discharged home. After reviewing the discharge instructions with Mrs. Granger, which of the following statements indicates to the LPN/LVN that further teaching is needed?

(A) "I am going to cut back on milk and cream consumption and start eating other dairy products instead."
(B) "I'm going to remove coffee and any food or drinks that contain caffeine from my diet."
(C) "I will make aspirin my pain reliever of choice."
(D) "I'm scheduled to go to a smoking cessation group this Tuesday."

Physiological Integrity:
Reduction of Risk Potential

Q–37

A neonate is delivered after a full-term pregnancy with an intact omphalocele. Which of the following is NOT an intervention for the management of the omphalocele prior to surgical repair?

(A) Apply saline-soaked pads to the sac.
(B) Insert a nasogastric tube.
(C) Cover the defect and the abdomen in a plastic wrap.
(D) Offer a pacifier to the infant.

Answers

(C) Aspirin irritates the mucosal lining of the gastrointestinal tract and is not recommended for use by clients with peptic ulcer disease, making answer (C) correct. It is suggested to clients with peptic ulcer disease to avoid a diet rich in milk and cream, which stimulate acid secretion. Foods and beverages with caffeine increase acid secretion. Coffee, even decaffeinated forms, stimulates acid secretion also. Smoking causes decreased secretion of bicarbonate into the duodenum from the pancreas. Bicarbonate decreases the acidity in the GI tract. Therefore, clients with PUD should be encouraged to stop smoking.

(D) Omphalocele is the herniation of abdominal contents through the umbilical cord ring. Protection from infection and rupture of the sac are vitally important to the infant's safety prior to repair. Wrapping the sac in saline-soaked pads keeps the area moist, which helps prevent infection. Covering the sac with saline pads and wrapping the abdomen with plastic wrap help protect the defect. A nasogastric tube is inserted to decompress the gastrointestinal tract and reduce the bowel. The correct answer is (D). A pacifier is offered after surgery for oral gratification.

Physiological Integrity:
Physiological Adaptation

Q–38

Mrs. Strachand was severely burned in an automobile accident. The burns cover her entire anterior chest and right arm. Using the Rule of Nines, the LPN/LVN would calculate the body surface area (BSA) that is burned to be

(A) 9%
(B) 18%
(C) 27%
(D) 36%

Physiological Integrity:
Reduction of Risk Potential

Q–39

While looking over a client's laboratory findings, the day shift LPN/LVN notices that the serum potassium of the client is 4.1 mEq/L. Which of the following is the most appropriate nursing action after discovering this information?

(A) Document this normal finding in the medical record.
(B) Call the physician immediately for an order to increase this dangerously low potassium level.
(C) Check that the client is oriented. This reading is critically high and could cause confusion.
(D) This value is a little low. Encourage the client to drink 12 oz of orange juice and eat a banana to increase the serum potassium level.

Answers

(C) The Rule of Nines is a method that uses percentages to calculate the amount of body surface area (BSA) that has been burned. The body is divided into nine sections, each calculated as a percentage that is a multiple of nine. Together, the head and neck make up 9% of the BSA. Each arm is 9% of the BSA. Each leg is 18% of the BSA. The anterior chest is 18% of the BSA. The posterior chest (including the back and buttocks) is 18% of the BSA. The perineum, the only exception to the "nine" rules, is 1% of the BSA. Using this information, the correct answer is 27%, or answer (C). The right arm is 9% and the anterior chest is 18%.

(A) The normal range for serum potassium is 3.8 to 5.0 mEq/L. The client's potassium level is within normal range. The correct nursing action would be to document this finding, answer (A). There is no need for the physician to be notified immediately, and further interventions are not necessary for a normal finding.

Physiological Integrity:
Pharmacological Therapies

Q–40

The LPN/LVN is preparing to administer Vancomycin 1 gram mixed in 500 mL of IV solution. The medication is to be administered over 90 minutes. At what rate should the medication be set at in drops per minute with a drop factor of 15 gtt/mL?

(A) 15 gtt/min
(B) 33 gtt/min
(C) 56 gtt/min
(D) 83 gtt/min

Physiological Integrity:
Physiological Adaptation

Q–41

Follow a drop of blood as it circulates through the right side of the heart, using all of the following cardiac structures:

(A) Tricuspid valve
(B) Vena cava
(C) Right ventricle
(D) Right atrium
(E) Pulmonic valve
(F) Pulmonary artery

A–40

(D) The formula to calculate this problem is: x gtt/min = volume/time (in minutes) × drop factor.

$$x \frac{\text{gtt}}{\text{min}} = \frac{\text{volume}}{\text{time}}$$

x gtt/min = 83

The correct answer is (D).

A–41

(B), (D), (A), (C), (E), (F). The blood enters the right atrium of the heart via the superior vena cava. From the right atrium, blood goes through the tricuspid valve to the right ventricle. The blood then continues out of the right side of the heart into the pulmonary artery by way of the pulmonic valve.

Physiological Integrity:
Reduction of Risk Potential

Q–42

Mr. Greene is a client in a long-term nursing facility who requires tube feedings via his PEG (percutaneous endoscopic gastrostomy) tube. Which of the following would the LPN/LVN know to watch for as the most common complication of tube feedings?

(A) Constipation
(B) Loose, watery stools
(C) Vomiting
(D) Excessive belching

Physiological Integrity:
Physiological Adaptation

Q–43

Which of the following pathogens is most commonly found in an infection of the bladder and urinary tract?

(A) *Streptococcus pyogenes* (Group A Strep)
(B) *Salmonella*
(C) *Staphylococcus aureus* (*S. aureus*)
(D) *Eschericha coli* (*E. coli*)

Answers

(B) The most frequent complication of tube feedings, whether through nasogastric or PEG (percutaneous endoscopic gastrostomy) tube, is diarrhea or loose, watery stools. This is a reaction caused by intolerance to the formula solution or the rate that the formula is being given. Constipation can occur any time food is passed through the gastrointestinal tract, but it is not the most common condition caused by tube feedings. Vomiting could also indicate intolerance to the tube feeding rate, but it is less common than diarrhea. Belching is not a side effect known to be caused by tube feeding.

(D) The correct answer is *Eschericha coli* (*E. coli*), (D). *Streptococcus pyogenes* (Group A Strep) and *Staphylococcus aureus* (*S. aureus*) are pathogens commonly found in the upper respiratory tract, the skin, and the hair. *Salmonella* is found in the lower gastrointestinal tract.

Physiological Integrity:
Physiological Adaptation

Q–44

The physician diagnoses a client with septicemia. Which of the following assessment findings would support this diagnosis?

(A) Bilateral knee pain
(B) Reddened tissue surrounding an injury site
(C) Drainage from an injury site
(D) Temperature of 101° F

Psychosocial Integrity

Q–45

A male client with diagnosed bipolar disorder is hospitalized on the psychiatric unit. At a community activity, the client becomes disruptive and is seen flirting with female clients. Which of the following is the most appropriate intervention for this behavior?

(A) Pull the client aside to remind him of the unit rules and set boundaries for his behavior.
(B) Tell the other clients to ignore the flirtatious actions of the male client.
(C) Avert the attention of the male client and lead him to his room.
(D) Have the client return to his room immediately because of his inappropriate behavior.

Answers

A–44

(D) Septicemia is the invasion of pathogenic bacteria into the blood stream. Symptoms of septicemia include temperature elevation, backache, headache, elevated pulse, elevated respiratory rate, nausea, vomiting, diarrhea, chills, and general malaise. The correct answer is (D), temperature of 101° F. Pain, redness, or drainage from an injury site suggests local, rather than systemic, infection or inflammation.

A–45

(C) The most appropriate response to this behavior would be to avoid confronting and/or threatening the client while removing the inappropriate behavior. Distraction is a good approach to ease removal of the client, making answer (C) correct. Averting the client's attention and escorting him to his room is neither confrontational nor threatening. Pulling the client aside and/or reprimanding him, as in answers (A) and (D), are both confrontational and threatening to a client. This could cause agitation. Having the other clients ignore the behavior will not remove the potentially hazardous situation.

Q–46

The nursing assistant runs out of a hospital room yelling that the patient fell to the floor. The LPN/LVN is rehearsing in her mind the order of nursing actions that should be performed when at the client's side. Arrange the following into the correct order of priority, with the highest-priority action listed first:

(A) Assess airway patency.
(B) Assess for injury.
(C) Move the client into bed.
(D) Check heart rate and blood pressure.
(E) Call the client's physician.

Q–47

Which of the following are conditions associated with Cushing's syndrome? Select all that apply.

(A) Easy bruising
(B) Buffalo hump
(C) Hyperglycemia
(D) Excessive scalp hair growth
(E) Hyponatremia
(F) Trunk obesity

Answers

The correct order is: **(A)**, **(D)**, **(B)**, **(C)**, and **(E)**. Assessing airway patency is the primary concern upon initiating emergency actions. If the airway is obstructed, CPR steps would be continued (i.e., Heimlich maneuver, rescue breathing, chest compressions, etc.). If the airway is patent, cardiopulmonary stability is measured by checking all vital signs. Once cardiopulmonary status is stable, the client can be assessed for any injuries caused by the fall. Moving the client to bed is not a top priority above assessing cardiopulmonary status. If the client could be further injured during the transfer process, this should be avoided until the safest transfer method is available. The physician should be notified of the fall, client's status, and any injuries once assessment and necessary interventions have been initiated.

Answers **(A)**, **(B)**, **(C)**, and **(F)** should all be selected. Clinical manifestations associated with Cushing's syndrome include: easy bruising, moon face, buffalo hump, hyperglycemia, hypokalemia, sodium retention, hypertension, truncal obesity, thin extremities, thinning of scalp hair, increased body and facial hair, acne, muscle wasting, poor wound healing, and mood changes. Excessive scalp hair growth and hyponatremia are not associated with Cushing's syndrome.

Health Promotion and Maintenance

Q-48

A client visiting the physician's office for an annual physical is about to perform a visual acuity test using the Snellen chart. Which statement is most accurate when explaining the examination to the client?

(A) "This exam tests your ability to read small print from a close distance."
(B) "This exam tests your peripheral vision."
(C) "This exam tests your ability to see colors."
(D) "This exam tests your visual acuity from far distances."

Physiological Integrity:
Physiological Adaptation

Q-49

Which of the following is the most important information obtained from a client that presents to the physician's office with right calf tenderness?

(A) High levels of work-related stress
(B) Use of oral contraceptives
(C) Left femur fracture 18 months prior
(D) Plays in a soccer league

Answers

(D) The visual acuity exam involving the Snellen chart tests long-distance vision. The client is asked to read letters from 20 feet away. The letters become consecutively smaller progressing down the chart. Jaeger's chart is used to test close distant vision. A tangent screen is used to test peripheral vision by gradually bringing an object into peripheral view and having the patient indicate when they see an object in their field of vision. Ishihara's plates are used to test for color vision.

(B) The client is displaying a characteristic symptom of a DVT (deep vein thrombosis). DVTs are dangerous as they can lead to pulmonary emboli if the thrombus becomes mobile and travels to the lungs. Risk factors for developing a DVT include: history of varicose veins, cardiovascular disease, pregnancy, oral contraceptive use, immobility, or recent surgery/injury. Stress is not a factor associated with a DVT. An injury 18 months ago is no longer a threat for developing a DVT. Playing soccer could cause shin splints, which would cause calf tenderness. However, a DVT should be ruled out before any other explanation is given for the calf tenderness.

Health Promotion and Maintenance

Q–50

Ms. Winters is visiting the pediatrician with her newborn baby girl, Emily. Ms. Winters has breastfed Emily since birth and wonders when Emily will be able to eat other foods. What age is the earliest that introduction of other foods into the infant's diet could begin?

Health Promotion and Maintenance

Q–51

Mrs. Foster thinks she might be pregnant and visits the physician's office. A urine sample pregnancy test is performed. The elevation of which of the following hormones in the urine would indicate that Mrs. Foster is indeed pregnant?

(A) Human growth hormone (hGH)
(B) Human chorionic gonadotropin (hCG)
(C) Estrogen
(D) Oxytocin

Answers

A-50

ANSWER: Four months
RATIONALE: Until four months of age, breast milk provides the nutrients necessary for infant growth and metabolism. Infant rice cereal is recommended as the first food to introduce. Any food introduced any earlier than four months might be dangerous to the infant's developing gastrointestinal system.

A-51

(B) Human chorionic gonadotropin (hCG) is released by the trophoblast, outer cell layer of the developing fetus in the zygote stage. hCG can be detected in the blood and urine as early as 10 to 14 days after conception, indicating early pregnancy. Human growth hormone (hGH) is responsible for the growth of bones, muscles, and other organs. Estrogen is important for maintaining pregnancy, but it is not used to diagnose pregnancy. Estrogen elevation does not occur until the seventh week of gestation. Oxytocin promotes uterine contractility and the stimulation of milk ejection from the breasts. During pregnancy oxytocin assists the labor process that results in birth.

Health Promotion and Maintenance

Q–52

During her visit to the clinic, testing is performed that confirms Mrs. Foster's suspected pregnancy. Mrs. Foster states that her last menstrual period (LMP) began on March 12. Using Nägele's rule, what would the LPN/LVN calculate Mrs. Foster's estimated date of confinement (EDC) to be?

(A) December 11 of that year
(B) January 2 of the following year
(C) December 27 of that year
(D) December 19 of that year

Physiological Integrity:
Pharmacological Therapies

Q–53

Two days ago the physician prescribed changes to the insulin regimen of a diabetic client. The new regimen involves the following order:

Humulin $\frac{70}{30}$ 15 units sc BID at 9:00

At midnight the client complains of "not feeling right." The client's skin is cool and clammy. Which of the following nursing actions is appropriate for the LPN/LVN assigned to the client to include in the client's care for the next 24 hours?

(A) Encourage an hs snack.
(B) Hold the A.M. insulin dose.
(C) Decrease the A.M. insulin dose to 10 units.
(D) Give the client Humulin R insulin instead of Humulin $\frac{70}{30}$.

Answers

(D) Nägele's rule calculates the estimated date of confinement (EDC) using the following formula: the first day of the last normal menstrual period (LMP) minus three months, plus seven days, plus one year. Three months before the date of Mrs. Foster's LMP is December 12 of the previous year. December 12 plus 7 days is December 19 of the previous year. Therefore, the EDC is December 19 of that year, answer (D).

(A) Encouraging an hs (hour of sleep) snack will help avoid hypoglycemia in the middle of the night caused from peaking effects of the P.M. insulin dose. Without a written physician's order, a nurse may not adjust the prescribed amount or dosage of a medication. Holding or decreasing the A.M. insulin dose will not affect hypoglycemia that occurs at midnight. Humulin R is regular insulin. Regular insulin is fast-acting. Humulin $\frac{70}{30}$ contains a 70% to 30% mixture of NPH (intermediate-acting) insulin to Humulin R (regular or fast-acting) insulin. Giving 15 units of regular insulin alone without a serum glucose that can sustain the effects of the dose can be fatal to a client.

Physiological Integrity:
Pharmacological Therapies

Q–54

Prescription of which of the following medications to a client with glaucoma should alert the LPN/LVN to clarify the order with the physician prior to administration?

(A) Nalbuphine (Nubain)
(B) Aspirin
(C) Benazepril (Lotensin)
(D) Atropine sulfate (Sal-Tropine)

Physiological Integrity:
Physiological Adaptation

Q–55

Mr. Sanders, an 83-year-old client, presents to the clinic complaining of a persistent "whistling sound" in his ears. How would the LPN/LVN document this complaint in the medical record?

Answers

(D) Glaucoma is a condition of the eye that involves an increase in intraocular pressure. Untreated glaucoma can lead to permanent blindness. Use of atropine sulfate (Sal-Tropine) causes pupil dilation, which can obstruct the drainage of aqueous humor from the eye and lead to an acute attack of increased intraocular pressure. Nalbuphine (Nubain) is an opioid analgesic. Nubain does not affect intraocular pressure. The use of aspirin for any therapeutic effect is not contraindicated for clients with glaucoma. Benazepril (Lotensin) is used to lower blood pressure in hypertensive patients. Benazepril (Lotensin) is safe for use by clients with glaucoma as well.

ANSWER: Tinnitus
RATIONALE: Tinnitus is defined as a sound heard in one or both ears. The sound could be described as ringing, buzzing, or whistling, and occurs without an external stimulus. Causes of tinnitus include an ear infection, side effects of certain medications, a blockage in the eustachian tube, or an injury to the head. Further assessment and patient history should be reviewed to determine the cause of the client's symptom.

Physiological Integrity:
Reduction of Risk Potential

Q–56

The LPN/LVN is preparing for a sterile procedure that requires using sterile 4 × 4 gauze. Which of the following would indicate contamination of the open 4 × 4s?

(A) The LPN/LVN pours sterile saline onto the sterile 4 × 4s that are sitting on the bedside table.

(B) The LPN/LVN opens the 4 × 4s just prior to use to avoid prolonged air exposure.

(C) The 4 × 4s remain within sterile packaging borders on a bedside table that is positioned at or above waist level.

(D) The 4 × 4s are picked up with sterile forceps.

Safe and Effective Care Environment:
Safety and Infection Control

Q–57

Which of the following would be the most appropriate room assignment for a child with lymphocytic leukemia who is being admitted to the unit?

(A) A semiprivate room with another child with leukemia

(B) A semiprivate room with a child who is diagnosed with FUO

(C) A private room on the pediatric medical floor

(D) A private room in the intensive care unit

Answers

(A) Keeping the 4 × 4s within sterile packaging borders on a surface that is at or above waist level and avoiding prolonged exposure to air are principles used to maintain sterility of equipment and supplies. To prevent contamination, the 4 × 4s should not be touched with any materials that have failed to maintain sterile technique themselves. It is proper to use sterile forceps or hands with properly applied sterile gloves to move sterile 4 × 4s while maintaining sterility. The correct answer (A) allows contamination through capillary action of the 4 × 4s. As the saline solution contacts the surface of the bedside table, the sterility is compromised because bacteria from the table travel through the fluid to contact the 4 × 4s.

(C) Until the degree of leukemia involvement is determined in the child, it is best to keep the child away from other children as much as possible. The white blood cells of a client with leukemia are ineffective. This causes decreased immunity. Infection from another child or person could be detrimental to a child with this condition. A semiprivate room is not recommended at this time. Unless the child is in critical condition, assignment to an intensive care bed is not necessary.

Health Promotion and Maintenance

Q–58

A physician schedules a client for a stress electrocardiogram. The client asks the LPN/LVN why this test is needed. The most accurate explanation from the nurse would be:

(A) "The test will determine the heart rate you want to achieve during exercise."
(B) "The doctor will be able to tell how much exercise you need to add to your daily routine in order to stay healthy."
(C) "The doctor is looking to see how exercise affects your heart."
(D) "The test will tell if you are likely to suffer from a heart attack in the next year."

Safe and Effective Care Environment:
Coordinated Care

Q–59

The nurse is caring for a client diagnosed with cancer. The healthcare provider recently told the client that there is no further treatment available for the cancer and the client's life expectancy was limited to a few weeks. The client suddenly stops breathing and the nurse is aware that there is no do-not-resuscitate order on the client's chart. What is the nurse's best action?

(A) Immediately call the healthcare practitioner for a do-not-resuscitate order.
(B) Begin performing CPR on the client.
(C) Call the client's family and request their input about further treatment.
(D) Wait two minutes and reassess the client.

Answers

A–58

(C) A stress electrocardiogram monitors the heart while the client progressively increases exercise levels. The physician will read the electrocardiogram, a graph of the client's heart function, to determine if cardiac dysfunction occurred during the exercise. The correct answer is (C). The physician is looking to see how the stress of exercise affects the client's heart. The "target heart rate" or rate that the client should reach during normal exercise is determined based on the client's age and gender. The test may indicate if a client needs to alter his/her daily exercise routine, but this is not the purpose of performing the test. An ECG will not determine the likelihood of a client suffering from a heart attack.

A–59

(B) Unless a client has a do-not-resuscitate order on the chart, the nurse (or any healthcare professional) is obligated to begin CPR. The nurse cannot wait and perform any other action except to begin CPR.

Physiological Integrity:
Physiological Adaptation

Q–60

Mr. Dwindell is admitted to the unit with severe dehydration caused by persistent nausea, vomiting, and diarrhea. Which of the following fluids would the physician most likely start the client on?

(A) 0.45% sodium chloride with added potassium
(B) 0.9% sodium chloride with added potassium
(C) 3% sodium chloride with added potassium
(D) 0.9% sodium chloride

Physiological Integrity:
Physiological Adaptation

Q–61

J. Cramer is a 17-year-old client with sickle cell anemia. Which of the following is NOT a common treatment and care modality for a client with this condition?

(A) Pain management
(B) Preventing infection
(C) Fluid restriction
(D) Red blood cell transfusions

Answers

(A) The client in this case needs a hypotonic solution to help the dehydrated cells pull in and regain fluid. 0.45% sodium chloride or $\frac{1}{2}$ normal saline is an example of a hypotonic solution. Potassium is lost along with the body fluids expelled through diarrhea and vomiting. Adding this to the fluid solution will replenish the body with this essential electrolyte. The correct answer is (A). 0.9% sodium chloride or normal saline is an isotonic solution. The constituents in isotonic solutions are similar to the fluid in the blood. Using this type of solution would not change the dehydrated state since it will not add or remove fluid from the body cells. 3% sodium chloride is a hypertonic solution. Using a hypertonic solution would lead to further dehydration by pulling fluid from the cells.

(C) Acute pain can be very severe during a sickle cell crisis due to hypoxia caused by inadequate blood flow to various tissues or organs. Pain management during crisis includes analgesics, relaxation techniques, and distraction. Techniques are used to prevent reoccurrence of symptoms once acute pain is controlled. Clients with sickle cell anemia are unusually susceptible to infection. Fluid is encouraged for sickle cell clients in order to promote dilution of the blood, which prevents clumping of sickled cells. Answer (C) is the correct choice. Red blood cell transfusions are common therapy used to prevent complications from sickle cell anemia.

Safe and Effective Care Environment:
Safety and Infection Control

Q–62

Mrs. Stanley is a neutropenic client in the medical unit of the hospital. As the lunch trays are being passed out, the LPN/LVN would carefully examine the foods on the tray to be sure they are appropriate for the client. Which of the following would NOT need to be removed from the tray by the LPN/LVN prior to bringing the tray into the room?

(A) Garden salad with packaged low sodium dressing
(B) Celery with bleu cheese dressing
(C) Apple slices
(D) Canned peach halves

Safe and Effective Care Environment:
Coordinated Care

Q–63

The physician has written an order for a client to be weighed daily. Which of the following instructions provided by the LPN/LVN to the nursing assistant is most important for obtaining accurate daily results?

(A) The client should be weighed at the same time every day.
(B) The client should not have had anything to eat or drink for 30 minutes prior to weighing.
(C) The client should remove slippers from their feet prior to being weighed.
(D) If using an internal bed scale, it is important to subtract 5 lbs from the results to account for the linens on the bed.

A–62

(D) Neutropenia is a condition where the number of circulating white blood cells (WBCs) in the client's blood is decreased. The risk for infection is very high for clients with this condition. Raw fruits and vegetables may be contaminated with microbes and should not be included in the diet of a neutropenic client. Garden salad, celery, and apples are all raw vegetables. Thoroughly cooked or canned fruits and vegetables are considered safe for a client with neutropenia. The correct choice is (D), canned peach halves.

A–63

(A) In order to obtain the most accurate results, a client should be weighed at the same time every day. Eating or drinking prior to weighing should not dramatically affect the results. The same amount of clothing should be worn with each daily reading. If an internal bed scale is used, the scale should be zeroed with the linens on the bed prior to the client getting into the bed. The same linens should be on the bed with each reading as were on the bed when the scale was zeroed. A bedside scale is zeroed prior to each use.

Q–64

The physician prescribes atorvastatin (Lipitor) for a client with elevated cholesterol levels that have not been sufficiently reduced with lifestyle changes. The LPN/LVN provides teaching about this medication to the client. Which of the following would the LPN/LVN explain as a potential side effect of taking this medication?

(A) Confusion
(B) Anemia
(C) Muscle pain
(D) Drowsiness

Q–65

The LPN/LVN is preparing to give a subcutaneous injection of Procrit 5,000 units. Which of the following needles would be appropriate for this type of injection?

(A) A $\frac{5}{8}$ inch, 25-gauge needle
(B) A 1 inch, 22-gauge needle
(C) A 1.5 inch, 25-gauge needle
(D) A 1.5 inch, 18-gauge needle

Answers

A–64

(**C**) Atorvastatin (Lipitor) is a lipid-lowering agent that lowers total and low-density lipoprotein (LDL) cholesterol in the body. Lipitor also helps increase high-density lipoprotein (HDL) cholesterol. The most common side effects associated with taking Lipitor include abdominal cramps, diarrhea, heartburn, and skin rashes. Other side effects that could be caused by taking Lipitor are joint pain (arthralgia) and muscle pain and weakness (myalagia). The correct answer is (C). Confusion, anemia, and drowsiness are not side effects that are associated with the use of Lipitor.

A–65

(**A**) An all-gauge needle is used to administer a subcutaneous injection to decrease the trauma caused by the needle puncture. The length of the needle selected for subcutaneous administration of a medication should be less than one inch, depending on the client's body mass. Needles most commonly come in $\frac{3}{8}$-inch and $\frac{5}{8}$-inch lengths. Answer (A) is correct because it is the only choice that has a needle length of less than 1 inch.

Physiological Integrity:
Physiological Adaptation

Q–66

A client is admitted to the unit with deep partial-thickness burns on bilateral lower extremities. The LPN/LVN knows that deep partial-thickness burns would exhibit which of the following characteristics?

(A) The burns involve the epidermis and dermis.
(B) The burns involve the epidermis, dermis, and subcutaneous tissue.
(C) The burns involve all skin layers and destruction of nerve endings.
(D) Necrosis is evident in the burned areas.

Physiological Integrity:
Physiological Adaptation

Q–67

The LPN/LVN is evaluating the arterial blood gas results of a client, which read as follows: pH = 7.30, $HCO_3^- = 26$ mEq/L, $PaCO_2 = 49$ mm Hg. Which of the following acid-base disturbances do these results represent?

(A) Respiratory alkalosis
(B) Metabolic alkalosis
(C) Respiratory acidosis
(D) Metabolic acidosis

Answers

(A) Deep partial-thickness burns involve the epidermis and dermis. The client will experience severe pain due to nerve injury, but the burns do not penetrate deep enough to destroy nerve endings. Vesicles will develop from deep burns. Superficial partial-thickness burns, such as sunburns, affect only the epidermis. Full-thickness burns involve the epidermis, dermis, and subcutaneous tissue, and destroy nerve endings. Necrosis is seen in full-thickness burns.

(C) These results represent respiratory acidosis, answer (C). Normal values for arterial blood pH are 7.35 to 7.45. Normal values for arterial blood HCO_3^- levels are 22 to 26 mEq/L. Normal values for $PaCO_2$ levels are 35 to 45 mm Hg. Respiratory acidosis is a disorder in which the arterial blood has a below normal pH and a higher than normal $PaCO_2$. HCO_3^- may be either normal or high. In respiratory alkalosis, arterial blood pH is high, $PaCO_2$ is low, and HCO_3^- may be either normal or low. In metabolic alkalosis, arterial blood pH is high, HCO_3^- is high, and $PaCO_2$ may be either normal or high. In metabolic acidosis, arterial blood pH is low, HCO_3^- is low, and $PaCO_2$ may be either normal or low.

Q–68

A client is on heparin therapy while being hospitalized for new onset atrial fibrillation. What laboratory test will the LPN/LVN check regularly to monitor the effects of this medication?

Q–69

A client is being discharged from the hospital after treatment for new onset atrial fibrillation. The client was started on warfarin (Coumadin). The LPN/LVN reviews the client's discharge instructions. Select all of the following foods that should be limited in a client's diet while on warfarin (Coumadin).

(A) Kale
(B) Spinach
(C) Green beans
(D) Broccoli
(E) Brussels sprouts
(F) Celery

Answers

ANSWER: Partial thromboblastin time (PTT)
RATIONALE: Heparin is an anticoagulant. It is used for clients who are at high risk for thrombus formation. In order to regulate the therapeutic levels of heparin, partial thromboblastin time (PTT) of the client's blood is tested periodically. PTT is the most accurate test for monitoring the effects of heparin therapy.

(A), (B), (C), (D), and **(E)** are correct. Warfarin is an anticoagulant used to prevent thromboembolic events for at-risk clients. Vitamin K reverses the effects of warfarin (Coumadin). Good dietary sources of vitamin K include green leafy vegetables (such as spinach, kale, and Brussels sprouts), broccoli, and green beans. With this considered, the only answer choice that is not a good source of vitamin K is answer (F). Celery contains very low amounts of vitamin K.

Physiological Integrity:
Pharmacological Therapies

Q–70

Mrs. Friedman, a client at the community clinic, has been diagnosed with tuberculosis (TB). Mrs. Friedman's medication regimen includes a combination of the medications rifampin (Rifadin) and isoniazid (INH). The client asks the LPN/LVN why she must take two medications for the same illness. Which of the following would be the most accurate response?

(A) "The rifampin (Rifadin) is given to minimize unpleasant side effects that isoniazid (INH) can cause."
(B) "When given together, the doses of each medication can be lowered to reduce the effects on the body."
(C) "Rifampin (Rifadin) kills the disease in your body and isoniazid (INH) will make sure that you cannot be infected with TB in the future."
(D) "Combining these medications keeps the TB from becoming a form that is resistant to treatment."

Physiological Integrity:
Physiological Adaptation

Q–71

Which of the following are symptoms associated with pernicious anemia? Select all that apply.

(A) Sore tongue
(B) Diarrhea and upset stomach
(C) Insomnia
(D) Paresthesias
(E) Arthralgia
(F) Weakness and fatigue

Answers

(**D**) If a single medication is used at one time, the tuberculosis pathogen can mutate to resist the medication. Combination therapy slows down this mutation process and allows the medications to be effective against the original TB pathogen. The correct answer is (D). One medication is not given to reduce or prevent side effects of the other medication. Both medications fight the TB pathogen. The medication doses are not changed when given in combination. Both medications fight the pathogen that is already existent in the body.

(**A**), (**B**), (**D**), and (**F**) are the correct answers. Pernicious anemia is an autoimmune disease in which the intestines are unable to absorb enough vitamin B_{12} to meet the needs of the body. Symptoms include the following: weakness and fatigue; tingling and numbness in the extremities (paresthesias); sore and reddened tongue; diarrhea, nausea, and vomiting; pallor; abdominal pain; confusion; and loss of proprioception (sense of position). Vitamin B_{12} is supplemented by means outside of the gastrointestinal tract to correct the deficiency. Insomnia and arthralgia (joint or bone pain) are not associated with pernicious anemia.

Physiological Integrity:
Physiological Adaptation

Q-72

A concerned mother brings her three-year-old son to the pediatric clinic after discovering a rash that started on his face and progressively spread down his entire body. The LPN/LVN describes the rash to the physician as pinpoint-sized reddened marks. Which of the following do these symptoms indicate that the child is infected with?

(A) Chicken pox
(B) Mumps
(C) Rubella
(D) Whooping cough

Physiological Integrity:
Pharmacological Therapies

Q-73

The physician has written an order for a client to receive 0.45% NaCl ($\frac{1}{2}$ normal saline) intravenously at a rate of 75 mL per hour. The drop factor of the tubing set is 20 drops per mL. The LPN/LVN should calculate the flow rate to be

(A) 20
(B) 25
(C) 50
(D) 75

Answers

(C) Rubella (German measles) involves a pinpoint rash that spreads quickly starting on the face and traveling down the body, answer (C). Chicken pox usually appears first on the trunk as well as the scalp. The rash is described as macular to papular in appearance, and the vesicles crust over. Mumps does not involve rash formation. Symptoms of mumps include fever, headache, malaise, and swollen salivary glands. Whooping cough or pertussis does not involve rash formation. Symptoms include coryza (inflammation of nasal mucosa), sneezing, watery eyes, cough that develops a "whooping" sound, fever, and vomiting.

(B) The formula to calculate this problem is: x gtt/min = volume/time (in minutes) × drop factor.

$$x \text{ gtt/min} = \frac{75 \text{ mL}}{60 \text{ min}} \times 20 \text{ gtt/min}$$

x Gtt/min = 25

The correct answer is (B).

Physiological Integrity:
Pharmacological Therapies

Q–74

Upon removing a breakfast tray from a room, the LPN/LVN calculates the client's intake. The client consumed the following: 4 oz of pudding, 6 oz of coffee, half of a 6-oz container of grape juice, and used 4 oz of milk over cold cereal. In milliliters, what should the nurse record as the client's intake for this meal?

(A) 480 mL
(B) 390 mL
(C) 510 mL
(D) 600 mL

Physiological Integrity:
Pharmacological Therapies

Q–75

Which of the following routes of administration takes effect most rapidly?

(A) IV
(B) IM
(C) PO
(D) Topical

Answers

A–74

(B) Oral fluid intake is being calculated. Oral fluid intake for this meal would include any consumed fluid or solid food that becomes liquid at room temperature. Pudding does not fit the category of oral fluid intake.

Oral Fluid Intake Calculation:

6 oz of coffee, 3 oz of grape juice, 4 oz of milk multiplied by 30 mL/oz = (6 + 3 + 4)30 = 390

The correct answer is (B), 390.

A–75

(A) The most rapid route of administration is intravenous (IV). IV administration puts the medication directly into the blood stream, which generally produces immediate effects. Intramuscular (IM) injection is slower than IV administration but becomes effective more quickly than other routes of administration. Oral (PO = by mouth) administration is the most common but often does not take effect quickly. Topical administration is usually the slowest route of administration.

Physiological Integrity:
Pharmacological Therapies

Q–76

The physician has prescribed promethazine (Phenergan) 12.5 mg IM q 4 hours prn for a chemotherapy client with severe nausea. The vial reads 50 mg of medication per mL of solution. How much solution should the LPN/LVN draw into the syringe for IM administration?

(A) 0.125 mL
(B) 0.25 mL
(C) 0.75 mL
(D) 1 mL

Physiological Integrity:
Physiological Adaptation

Q–77

A client with severe peptic ulcer disease undergoes a Billroth II surgical procedure. Which of the following best describes the alterations made to the gastrointestinal tract with this procedure?

(A) Antrectomy with anastomosis to the duodenum
(B) Antrectomy with anastomosis to the jejunum
(C) Vagus nerves are severed.
(D) Resection of the large bowel

Answers

(B) Solve for x mL using the following ratio method:

$$\frac{50 \text{ mg}}{1 \text{ mL}} = \frac{12.5 \text{ mg}}{x \text{ mL}}$$

$$50x = 12.5$$

$$x = \frac{12.5}{50}$$

$$x = 0.25 \text{ mL}$$

The correct answer is (B).

(B) Billroth II, also known as gastrojejunostomy, begins with the removal of the lower section of the antral portion of the stomach. This is the part of the stomach that secretes gastrin, which stimulates the secretion of gastric acid. A small portion of the duodenum and pylorus are also removed. The remaining stomach is then attached with an opening (anastomosed) to the jejunum of the small intestines. Answer (B) is correct. Answer (A) represents a Billroth I procedure. The severing of vagus nerves, answer (C), describes a vagotomy. Answer (D) describes a colon resection.

Q–78

The LPN/LVN has assigned an unlicensed assistive personnel (UAP) to change the linens on a client's bed. The LPN/
LVN will intervene if the UAP performs what action during
the linen change?

(A) The UAP puts on gloves before starting the linen change.
(B) The UAP places the clean linens on a clean towel in a chair
in the client's room.
(C) The UAP holds the soiled linens against the chest after
removing them from the bed.
(D) The UAP places the dirty linens in the linen receptacle in
the client's bathroom.

Physiological Integrity:
Physiological Adaptation

Q–79

Mr. Peters is admitted to the unit for a cardiac arrhythmia.
The LPN/LVN knows that this involves a malfunction in
the electrical conduction of the heart. Arrange the following
structures in the correct order to represent normal electrical
conduction of the heart.

(A) Atrioventricular (AV) node
(B) Bundle of His
(C) Bundle branches
(D) Purkinje fibers
(E) Sinoatrial (SA) node

A–78

(C) The LPN/LVN will intervene when the UAP places the dirty linens against a clean uniform. The other steps are appropriate during a linen change.

A–79

The correct order is (E), (A), (B), (C), and (D). Normal electrical conduction within the heart begins with stimulation of the sinoatrial (SA) node. The SA node is called the heart's pacemaker because it maintains the normal heart rate of 60 to 100 bpm for an adult. The SA node sends the electrical impulse to the AV node, which transmits the signal on through the bundle of His to the right and left bundle branches. The signal ends in the Purkinje fibers, located in the outside muscle layers of the heart.

Physiological Integrity:
Reduction of Risk Potential

Q–80

The LPN/LVN is evaluating a six-second long electrocardiogram (ECG) strip. Which of the following represents depolarization of the ventricular muscle?

(A) P wave
(B) T wave
(C) QRS complex
(D) PR interval

Physiological Integrity:
Physiological Adaptation

Q–81

Ms. Stafford comes to the clinic complaining of a severe headache and general malaise. Urinalysis results show hematuria. The client also has blood pressure of 169/92 and peripheral edema. Ms. Stafford visited the clinic two weeks ago with strep throat. Which of the following diagnoses do these findings best support?

(A) Acute glomerulonephritis
(B) Congestive heart failure
(C) Pulmonary edema
(D) Hypertensive encephalopathy

A–80

(**C**) Depolarization of the ventricular muscle of the heart is represented by the QRS complex on the electrocardiogram (ECG) strip. The correct answer is (C). The P wave represents atrial depolarization. The T wave represents ventricle muscle repolarization. The PR interval is the distance from the beginning of the P wave to the center of the R wave in the QRS complex. This interval represents the time used to stimulate the SA node, depolarize the atria, and conduct the impulse through the AV node prior to ventricular depolarization.

A–81

(**A**) Glomerulonephritis is inflammation of the capillaries of the glomeruli of the kidneys that often is preceded by a streptococcal infection, such as strep throat. This disease can be very vague and mild. However, symptoms can be very severe including hematuria, proteinuria, decreased urine output, fluid retention/edema, hypertension, headache, malaise, and flank pain. Fluid retention could lead to circulatory overload with dyspnea, engorged neck veins, cardiomegaly, and pulmonary edema. Acute glomerulonephritis may lead to serious conditions such as congestive heart failure (CHF), pulmonary edema, and hypertensive encephalopathy.

Q–82

Diuretics are often prescribed for treatment of acute glomer-ulonephritis to treat fluid overload and hypertension. Which of the following is least likely to be prescribed for this pur-pose in glomerulonephritis?

(A) Bumex
(B) Lasix
(C) Demadex
(D) Aldactone

Safe and Effective Care Environment:
Coordinated Care

Q–83

A nurse is working overnight on a very busy medical unit with one other nurse and two unlicensed personnel. About one hour into the shift, the first nurse smells alcohol on the breath of the second nurse and believes the nurse's speech is slightly slurred. What is the first nurse's best action in this situation?

(A) Recommend that the second nurse go into the lounge and drink coffee for 30 minutes.
(B) Call the nursing supervisor and report that the second nurse had become sick and needed to go home.
(C) Report the incident to the manager of the unit in the morning.
(D) Immediately inform the nursing supervisor that alcohol was noted on the second nurse's breath and that her speech appeared slurred.

Answers

A–82

(D) Loop diuretics are most commonly used to treat fluid overload and hypertension because of their effectiveness. Bumex, Lasix, and Demadex are all loop diuretics. Aldactone, a potassium-sparing diuretic, is very weak in comparison to loop diuretics. Answer (D) is the correct choice. Unless the client's potassium level is dangerously low, this medication is not usually prescribed. Sometimes potassium-sparing diuretics are used along with lower doses of other diuretics to help conserve the body's potassium levels.

A–83

(D) It is the nurse's responsibility to immediately notify a supervisor if there is a possibility that a coworker is impaired. The first nurse should not suggest that the nurse who smelled of alcohol go drink coffee because any possible chance of impairment must be reported to ensure client safety. It is not acceptable to lie for the nurse who is possibly impaired by telling the nurse to go home and then report the nurse as sick. Client safety is the most important thing for this nurse to think about at this time, so notification cannot wait until morning.

Health Promotion and Maintenance

Q–84

Education regarding testicular cancer is being provided to male clients at the primary care facility. It is recommended that males begin testicular self-examinations (TSE) at what age?

(A) 13 to 14 years old
(B) 17 to 18 years old
(C) 20 years old
(D) 40 years old

Health Promotion and Maintenance

Q–85

The LPN/LVN is teaching a male client how to perform a testicular self-examination (TSE). Which of the following is NOT accurate information for performing this procedure?

(A) "It is best to perform the exam in the shower."
(B) "The exam may hurt a little as you apply pressure to the testes."
(C) "Use your thumb and first two fingers to palpate the area."
(D) "If anything abnormal is detected, call your physician for further examination."

Answers

(A) Although testicular cancer is rare, the fatality rate of this type of cancer is very high. Testicular self-examination is recommended to all males starting from ages 13 to 14 and up. This is because testicular cancer is the most common cancer in young men (ages 15 to 35). A male with this type of cancer could be asymptomatic. Therefore, detection by palpation is necessary to provide early treatment. Answer (A) is correct.

(B) Testicular self-examinations should be performed once a month. The best place to perform the exam is in the shower, while the scrotal sac is warm and relaxed. Using the thumb and first two fingers, the testicles should be palpated. The testicle is movable and egg-shaped. Any lump, hard area, or enlargement of a testicle, whether painful or painless, should be reported to a physician. The correct answer is (B). The examination should be painless. If pain is experienced, too much pressure is being applied.

Psychosocial Integrity

Q–86

A 16-year-old female diagnosed with bulimia nervosa is admitted to an inpatient facility for psychiatric evaluation. Select all of the following that would be included in obtaining the client's initial assessment.

(A) Frequency of weighing
(B) Menstrual history
(C) Serum electrolyte values
(D) History of abuse
(E) Dieting patterns
(F) Use of diuretics
(G) Premorbid weight

Psychosocial Integrity

Q–87

Which of the following is a characteristic physical finding least likely to be found in clients with the eating disorder bulimia nervosa?

(A) Maintenance of a steady, normal weight
(B) Erosion of tooth enamel
(C) Loss of hair
(D) Electrolyte imbalance

Answers

All answer choices are correct. All of the information would be gathered about this client. Bulimia nervosa is an eating disorder characterized by binge eating followed by self-induced purging of the ingested substance. Clients with this condition may use emetics, diuretics, and/or laxatives chronically. This condition also involves an obsession with weight and appearance. During the initial exam of a client with bulimia nervosa, history regarding weight patterns, abuse, menstruation, dieting, and medication use will be gathered. Body language will be evaluated. Physical examination includes mental status evaluation and laboratory testing of electrolyte levels and complete blood count.

(C) Bulimia nervosa is a condition in which a client has an obsession with food and body weight. Clients with this disorder often binge on high-calorie foods and then experience a high amount of guilt that leads to purging of the food by self-inflicted vomiting or diarrhea. The cycle of binging and purging often leads to maintenance of a steady and normal weight. Due to frequent vomiting episodes, clients with this disorder often have eroded tooth enamel and multiple dental caries from contact with acidic stomach contents. Electrolyte imbalances occur as a result of electrolyte loss caused by emesis and diarrhea. Hair loss caused by malnutrition is commonly seen in clients with anorexia nervosa, a condition that involves complete food aversion. Answer (C) is correct.

Psychosocial Integrity

Q–88

The LPN/LVN at a clinic answers a phone call from an 18-year-old rape victim. The nurse tells the victim to go to the emergency room for a medical examination. Which of the following additional instructions for the victim is of highest priority?

(A) Gather belongings that might be necessary for a short hospital stay.
(B) Write down every remembered detail from the incident.
(C) Call a support person immediately.
(D) Do not take a shower before going to the hospital.

Psychosocial Integrity

Q–89

A client is hospitalized due to complications of lung cancer two weeks after initial diagnosis. The client's husband frequently yells at the LPN/LVN and staff as they perform necessary and normal actions. Which of the following is the best response to this behavior from the nurse?

(A) Kindly ask the husband to act more appropriately or he may need to leave the facility.
(B) Understand that anger is a normal response to this type of circumstance and offer support as the husband works through his grief.
(C) Tell the husband that being angry is not going to make the disease go away.
(D) Report the behavior to the charge nurse and ask for an assignment change.

Answers

(D) Rape is any form of sexual violence or assault inflicted on an unwilling victim. A thorough physical exam will be performed at the hospital. Evidence may only be available on the victim or the victim's clothes. The victim should be advised not to shower, brush teeth, drink or eat, douche, change clothes, or manipulate any surface or body orifice that could contain evidence against the perpetrator. The victim can wait to tell the details of the incident to medical professionals at the hospital as opposed to writing them down. Gathering belongings and/or calling a support person may be helpful, but these actions are not high priorities in this situation.

(B) The husband of this client is experiencing grief from the thought of losing his wife very soon. These behaviors represent the client in the anger stage of the grieving process. The reaction from the nurse should be to understand that the husband's anger is a normal response to feelings of loss and help him move through the grieving process. Withdrawal or retaliation should be avoided, and the staff should not take the behavior personally. Other responses that might help a person in this circumstance would be to help him deal with any underlying needs, provide structure and security, and allow as much control as possible over the situation.

Psychosocial Integrity

Q–90

The LPN/LVN assigned to a homosexual male is responsible for relaying positive HIV test results to the client. Which of the following responses would the nurse expect initially?

(A) Disbelief
(B) Acceptance
(C) Anger
(D) Depression

Psychosocial Integrity

Q–91

A client with obsessive-compulsive disorder (OCD) is admitted to the psychiatric facility for treatment. Select all of the following that are included in medical treatment of this disorder.

(A) Prescription of selective serotonin reuptake inhibitors (SSRIs)
(B) Behavior therapy
(C) Prescription of benzodiazepines
(D) Imagery
(E) Distraction
(F) Electroconvulsive therapy (ECT)

Answers

(A) Initial response to receiving sad or bad news is disbelief or denial, answer (A). Grief is a normal response to loss or feelings of powerlessness. When people experience grief, they must work through stages of changing emotions, which usually progress as follows: disbelief, anger, bargaining, depression, and eventually acceptance.

(A) and **(B)** are correct. Treatment of obsessive-compulsive disorder (OCD) includes use of selective serotonin reuptake inhibitors (SSRIs) and behavior therapy. OCD is thought to be caused partially by low levels of serotonin in the brain. SSRIs increase serotonin levels. Behavior therapy involves exposure to a feared object or situation and prevention of carrying out compulsive behavior. Benzodiazepines are not prescribed to treat OCD. Imagery and distraction are relaxation techniques usually used as pain relief methods. Electroconvulsive therapy is used to treat severe depression when other treatment modalities are ineffective.

Q–92

Valium is a type of benzodiazepine. Which of the following is NOT a prescriptive use of benzodiazepines?

(A) Treatment of seizures
(B) Muscle relaxant
(C) Treatment of anxiety
(D) Treatment of psychosis

Q–93

An inpatient client at the psychiatric facility is placed on Haldol for treatment of a psychotic disorder. Which of the following client symptoms should be immediately reported to the physician?

(A) Dizziness
(B) Tremors
(C) Sensitivity to light
(D) Constipation

Answers

A-92

(D) Psychosis, a mental disorder that involves a severe loss of contact with reality, is treated with neuroleptic medications such as Haldol and Risperdal. The correct answer is (D). Treatment of seizures, skeletal muscle relaxation, and treatment of anxiety are all valid uses for benzodiazepines.

A-93

(B) Muscle tremors are a type of serious adverse effects, known as extrapyramidal effects, that can occur from neuroleptic drug use. These effects are caused by nerve impulses traveling outside of the normal tracts of the central nervous system. Extrapyramidal side effects include muscular rigidity, tremors, bradykinesia, and difficulty walking. These symptoms often make the client appear to have Parkinson's disease. The physician should be immediately notified if these symptoms appear. Dizziness, sensitivity to light, and constipation are all common, manageable side effects of neuroleptic drug use.

Physiological Integrity:
Pharmacological Therapies

Q–94

A manic-depressive client is placed on Lithium. The LPN/LVN provides instruction to the client regarding this medication. Which of the following is an appropriate statement by the nurse regarding this medication?

(A) "You will need to restrict fluid intake while on this medication."
(B) "You may skip your dose if you feel well when you wake up in the morning."
(C) "You will need to visit your doctor regularly for laboratory blood testing."
(D) "This medication may cause you to lose weight. So be sure to eat enough throughout the day."

Physiological Integrity:
Pharmacological Therapies

Q–95

A client on Lithium for antimanic effects comes to the clinic for regular testing of serum Lithium level. Which of the following indicates a therapeutic level of this medication in the blood?

(A) 0.45 mEq/L
(B) 0.78 mEq/L
(C) 1.6 mEq/L
(D) 2.0 mEq/L

A-94

(C) Lithium is a medication used to decrease or prevent acute manic episodes. To ensure therapeutic effects and prevent toxicity, a client on this medication will need to have regular serum Lithium levels drawn. Initially this test is drawn twice weekly. Once therapeutic levels are reached, the test is performed every two to three months. While on this medication, a client is informed to drink a lot of fluid and consume a moderate amount of sodium in the diet. This prevents low sodium levels, which can lead to Lithium toxicity. The client should be instructed never to skip a dose in order to maintain therapeutic levels. Weight gain, not weight loss, is a side effect of this medication.

A-95

(B) The range that indicates therapeutic serum Lithium level is 0.5 to 1.5 mEq/L, answer (B). Any level below this range may not be producing desired effects. A level higher than this is toxic and lethal to a client. Answer (A), 0.45 mEq/L, is below therapeutic range. The client's Lithium dosage should be increased. Answers (C) and (D) indicate toxic levels of Lithium. The medication should be held, and the client should be monitored closely for adverse effects.

Safe and Effective Care Environment:
Safety and Infection Control

Q–96

An 11-year-old child is experiencing seizure activity. When reporting the event in the medical record, the LPN/LVN would record all of the following in the medical record, except

(A) time of seizure onset
(B) duration of the seizure
(C) demographic data of the client
(D) position of extremities before, during, and after the seizure

Physiological Integrity:
Physiological Adaptation

Q–97

The LPN/LVN walks into the room just prior to the client suddenly becoming unconscious for approximately 20 seconds followed by uncontrolled jerking movements of the client's entire body. Which of the following types of seizures has the nurse just witnessed?

(A) Atonic seizure
(B) Tonic-clonic seizure
(C) Myoclonic seizure
(D) Absence seizure

Answers

(C) The nurse will need to record a description of events leading to the seizure activity, time of onset, duration of seizure activity, initial position of body parts (eyes, head, mouth, body, and extremities), any changes in position or lack thereof, skin characteristics, and facial expressions. These assessments will help in determining any details that contribute to or are associated with the client's seizure activity. The child's demographic data should be recorded elsewhere in the medical record and does not need to be repeated with every new entry. Answer (C) is correct.

(B) A seizure that begins with a loss of consciousness, usually including muscle stiffness, followed by jerking movements caused by alternating muscle contraction and relaxation is known as a tonic-clonic seizure, answer (B). Atonic seizures are characterized by sudden and momentary loss of muscle tone. Myoclonic seizures involve convulsive episodes followed by muscle contraction. Absence seizures involve brief loss of consciousness with little or no muscle tone changes.

Health Promotion and Maintenance

Q–98

An LPN/LVN is volunteering at the community clinic administering influenza vaccinations. Which of the following is the most important information to gather prior to administering the vaccine?

(A) Does the client have any allergy to eggs or egg products?
(B) Did the client receive an influenza vaccination last year?
(C) When was the last time the client received a pneumococcal vaccination?
(D) Has the client experienced flu-like symptoms following an influenza vaccination?

Physiological Integrity:
Pharmacological Therapies

Q–99

A client is receiving Robitussin 1200 mg q 12 hours for treatment of a productive cough associated with pneumonia. The bottle reads $\frac{100 \text{ mg}}{5 \text{ mL}}$. How many ounces would the client receive with each dose?

(A) 30
(B) 10
(C) 6
(D) 2

Answers

A–98

(A) Influenza vaccinations are made up of a small amount of the influenza virus administered via injection to promote antibody production and prevent development of the full-fledged viral infection. The virus is cultured in egg albumin. If a client is allergic to eggs or egg products, reaction to the albumin in the vaccine may be experienced. Answer (A) is correct. It is recommended for members of the general public to receive the influenza vaccine once a year. Pneumococcal vaccination, used to prevent bacterial pneumonia, does not interfere with influenza vaccination. It is common to experience mild flu-like symptoms following vaccination against influenza, as this vaccine is made from a strain of the influenza virus.

A–99

(D) $\frac{100 \text{ mg}}{5 \text{ mL}} = \frac{1200 \text{ mg}}{x \text{ mL}} = \frac{6000}{100} = 60$ mL. There are 30 mL per one ounce of fluid. $\frac{30 \text{ mL}}{1 \text{ oz}} = \frac{60 \text{ mL}}{x \text{ oz}} = \frac{60}{30} = 2$. Therefore, the client would receive 2 oz of Robitussin with each dose. The correct answer is (D).

Safe and Effective Care Environment:
Coordinated Care

Q–100

The nurse is caring for four clients who each want to leave the healthcare facility against medical advice. Which client may the nurse prevent from leaving?

(A) A 65-year-old client who states, "I'm tired of this place. I can get better at home."
(B) A 79-year-old client with abdominal pain who states, "I need a drink. I'm out of here."
(C) An 80-year-old client with dementia who is screaming and attempting to hit everyone.
(D) A 90-year-old client with heart failure who states, "If I'm going to die, it's going to be in my own bed."

Physiological Integrity:
Pharmacological Therapies

Q–101

A client complaining of constipation is prescribed lactulose (Cephulac) 20 g p.o. b.i.d. The nurse preparing the morning dose reads the constitution of medication to syrup solution as 10 g/15 mL. How many mL will the nurse prepare for the client?

(A) 10
(B) 15
(C) 20
(D) 30

Answers

(C) The nurse has the right to prevent someone from leaving a healthcare facility who is at risk of harming himself or others. None of the other clients meet this criteria.

(D) Solve for x mL using the following ratio method:

$$\frac{10 \text{ g}}{15 \text{ mL}} = \frac{20 \text{ g}}{x \text{ mL}}$$

$$10x = 300$$

$$x = \frac{300}{10}$$

$$x = 30 \text{ mL}$$

Answer (D) is correct.

Health Promotion and Maintenance

Q–102

The LPN/LVN is teaching Mr. Elbridge how to insert his new hearing aid. Arrange the following choices in the correct order for completing this task.

(A) Turn the hearing aid on and turn the volume up.
(B) Line up the earmold with the corresponding parts of the ear.
(C) Slightly rotate the earmold forward.
(D) Rotate the earmold backward.
(E) Insert the ear canal portion of the earmold.
(F) Turn the hearing aid off and the volume all the way down.

Health Promotion and Maintenance

Q–103

Mrs. Morris, age 67, has a history of colon cancer with no known metastasis. The cancer was removed surgically nine years ago and recurrence has not been identified since. When the client visits the community center for blood pressure screening, she tells the nurse that she has been suffering from constipation. Which of the following is the most appropriate response for the LPN/LVN to make?

(A) "You need to set up an appointment with your physician for evaluation."
(B) "Include 30 minutes of aerobic exercise in your daily routine."
(C) "Purchase an over-the-counter stool softener."
(D) "Let me give you a pamphlet on how to include more fiber in your diet."

Answers

A–102

(F), (B), (C), (E), (D), and **(A)** is the correct order of the answers. Prior to inserting the hearing aid, it should be turned off with the volume all of the way down. Next, locate the parts of the ear and the corresponding parts of the hearing aid and align them. Prior to inserting the ear canal portion of the earmold, it should be slightly rotated forward. As the earmold is guided into the ear canal, it is rotated backward. Once the earmold is snugly in place, turn the hearing aid on and adjust the volume according to the client's needs.

A–103

(A) Considering the client's history of colon cancer and the symptom she is experiencing, follow-up with her primary physician should be recommended. Constipation could be a sign of recurring malignancy in the bowel. Exercise, over-the-counter stool softener use, and increasing intake of dietary fiber are all suggestions to be given to someone experiencing constipation with no history or current conditions that could suggest a more serious complication.

Physiological Integrity:
Basic Care and Comfort

Q–104

A client with urinary incontinence is being introduced to possible non-pharmaceutical therapies to control this condition. The nurse describes a technique that is used to provide conscious control over body processes that at one time were considered involuntary. Which of the following therapies is being described?

(A) Biofeedback
(B) Progressive relaxation
(C) Imagery
(D) Hypnosis

Physiological Integrity:
Physiological Adaptation

Q–105

The nurse reviews the care plan of a post-op client after internal pacemaker placement. The LPN/LVN recognizes that the client is in the evaluation stage of the nursing process. Which of the following would NOT be an appropriate outcome to be expected from this client's plan of care?

(A) The client states that he will seek medical attention if he experiences palpitations.
(B) The client's white blood cell (WBC) count is 12,000/mm^3.
(C) Pulse is 60 to 70 BPM and regular.
(D) The client identifies the bulge in his chest as the pacemaker insertion site.

Answers

A-104

(A) Biofeedback, answer (A), teaches clients relaxation that allows dominance of parasympathetic responses over processes induced by the physiologic arousal during situations of stress. Progressive relaxation, commonly used for pain management, teaches a client to control physiologic responses to tension and anxiety. Imagery uses a client's mental images of an ideal state to produce self-healing and progress toward desired goals. Hypnosis uses concentration achieved through an altered state of consciousness to achieve desired effects.

A-105

(B) Expected outcomes following insertion of a pacemaker are signs that the site is free of infection, the client understands the self-care regimen, and the pacemaker is functioning properly. Indication by the client that he understands when to seek medical attention, such as with sudden heart rate changes, is an appropriate outcome. Identifying the bulge in his chest as the site covering the pacemaker device indicates appropriate understanding. A regular heart rate maintained between 60 and 90 BPM with no sudden changes suggests proper pacemaker function. Normal WBC count is 5,000 to 10,000/mm^3. In answer (B), the WBC count is elevated indicating infection, which is an inappropriate outcome.

Physiological Integrity:
Pharmacological Therapies

Q–106

A client is prescribed propantheline (Probanthel). Which of the following conditions would the nurse expect a client prescribed this medication to have?

(A) Congestive heart failure (CHF)
(B) Emphysema
(C) Peptic ulcer disease (PUD)
(D) Gout

Physiological Integrity:
Pharmacological Therapies

Q–107

The nurse provides teaching regarding pharmaceutical use of propantheline (Probanthel) to a client recently started on the medication. Which of the following would be an appropriate teaching point regarding side effects of Probanthel?

(A) Limit fluid intake.
(B) Maintain good oral hygiene.
(C) Avoid laxative use.
(D) Notify physician if a decrease in heart rate is noticed.

A–106

(C) Propantheline (Probanthel) is an antiulcer agent used to reduce signs and symptoms of peptic ulcer disease (PUD), answer (C). This medication decreases secretions in the gastrointestinal tract that result in irritation to the mucosal lining. Probanthel is not used in the treatment of congestive heart failure (CHF), emphysema, or gout.

A–107

(B) Side effects that are most frequently seen in clients on Probanthel include tachycardia, constipation, dry mouth, urinary hesitancy, and urinary retention. Suggestions for managing dry mouth include frequent oral rinses, chewing sugarless gum, sucking hard candy, and good oral hygiene. The client is encouraged to increase fluid and dietary fiber intake to relieve constipating effects of the medication. Use of laxatives may be necessary to prevent or treat constipation. An increase in heart rate is often noted as a side effect of this drug and should be reported to the physician if a high rate is experienced.

Physiological Integrity:
Physiological Adaptation

Q–108

A client is diagnosed with right-sided congestive heart failure (CHF). Select all of the following that are signs and symptoms associated with CHF of the right side of the heart.

(A) Dependent edema
(B) Pulmonary crackles
(C) Low oxygen saturation
(D) Distended neck veins
(E) Dyspnea
(F) Weight loss
(G) Cough

Physiological Integrity:
Physiological Adaptation

Q–109

A client is diagnosed with left-sided congestive heart failure (CHF). The client asks the nurse to explain what is going on with his heart. Which of the following is an accurate explanation of the defective mechanism?

(A) The right side of the heart is unable to pump effectively, leading to congestion of blood flow in the left side of the heart.
(B) The right side of the heart is pumping faster than the left side, which causes blood flow to back up in the left side of the heart.
(C) The flow of blood from the left side of the heart is obstructed by a clot in the aorta.
(D) The left side of the heart is unable to pump effectively, which leads to backup of the circulation in the lungs.

Answers

(A) and (D) are the correct answers. Clinical manifestations of right-sided congestive heart failure (CHF) include edema in the lower extremities or dependent edema, weight gain, enlarged liver, distended neck veins, accumulation of fluid in the peritoneal cavity called ascites, anorexia, nausea, nocturia, and weakness. Pulmonary crackles, low oxygen saturation, dyspnea, and cough are clinical manifestations of left-sided CHF. Weight loss is not seen in CHF of either side of the heart.

(D) Left-sided congestive heart failure (CHF) involves an inability of the left ventricle to pump effectively. This causes circulatory congestion in the left chambers of the heart. The blood that flows into the left ventricle comes from the lungs. Therefore, the congestion in the circulation in the left side of the heart causes blood to be backed up in the lungs as well. Answer (D) is correct. Answers (A), (B), and (C) are incorrect in explaining the mechanism that is malfunctioning in left-sided CHF.

Physiological Integrity:
Physiological Adaptation

Q–110

The nurse is developing the plan of care for a 20-year-old client with Crohn's disease. Which of the following would be an appropriate nursing diagnosis for this client?

(A) Ineffective breathing pattern
(B) Altered nutrition: less than body requirements
(C) Altered nutrition: more than body requirements
(D) Risk for fluid volume deficit

Physiological Integrity:
Physiological Adaptation

Q–111

The physician notes in the progress section of a female client's medical record that she has terminal insomnia. The LPN/LVN knows that this means the client

(A) is experiencing sleep deprivation to the point of being fatal.
(B) wakes up earlier than she wants to.
(C) has difficulty falling asleep.
(D) wakes up at frequent intervals in the night.

A–110

(**B**) Crohn's disease is an inflammatory bowel disease characterized by patches of inflammation through the full thickness of sections of the gastrointestinal tract. Symptoms include diarrhea, which may contain various amount of blood, and nutritional malabsorption. An appropriate nursing diagnosis would be altered nutrition: less than body requirements. Answer (B) is correct. Respiratory function is not commonly associated with this disorder. Altered nutrition: more than body requirements would more likely be assigned to a client with an overindulgent eating disorder. Fluid volume in the body is not normally a factor affected by this disorder.

A–111

(**B**) There are three types of insomnia. Initial insomnia refers to difficulty falling asleep. Intermittent insomnia is difficulty staying asleep due to frequent waking. Terminal insomnia involves premature waking. This type of insomnia involves the client waking early, feeling like more sleep is needed but unable to return to sleep. Answer (B) is correct. There is no recorded type of insomnia that refers to a critical level of sleep deprivation as described in answer (A).

Q–112

A 56-year-old male client is sent from the physician's office to be admitted to the hospital for a dangerously high blood pressure. The nurse obtains the client's medical history including the following home medications: labetalol, furosemide, and tamsulosin. The client tells the nurse that he stopped taking his medications two days ago because he was having sexual difficulties. This information leads the nurse to be most concerned with which of the following?

(A) The client is likely experiencing "rebound hypertension."
(B) The client needs to change to a different medication for treatment of prostate enlargement.
(C) The client should talk with his physician regarding sexual dysfunction.
(D) The client was incorrectly educated on the side effects of the prescribed medications.

Q–113

A client complains of photophobia and distorted vision when driving at night. What eye disorder is this client experiencing early symptoms of?

A–112

(A) A sudden stop in taking beta-blockers, such as labetolol, can lead to life-threatening hypertension called "rebound hypertension." This can also cause dangerous cardiac arrhythmias or myocardial ischemia. Of the answer choices, answer (A) includes the most important gathered information. Sexual dysfunction is a side effect of taking beta-blockers. The client should talk with the physician and follow instructions on how to prevent or diminish this effect from the medication. The client will need further instruction regarding side effects of the medications he is taking.

A–113

ANSWER: Cataracts
RATIONALE: Cataracts involve an increased opacity of the lens. Difficulty seeing in poor light or very bright light is an early sign of this change to the eye. Cataracts are usually a result of aging but can also be caused by trauma, intraocular disease, tobacco use, use of certain medications, or metabolic disorders. Cataracts can eventually lead to severely impaired vision or complete blindness.

Safe and Effective Care Environment:
Coordinated Care

Q–114

A client is scheduled to go for an electrophysiologic study (EPS). The doctor explains the procedure to the client and then asks the nurse to obtain written consent. The nurse should respond by

(A) telling the doctor that written consent needs to be obtained by the physician performing the procedure.
(B) informing the doctor that consent is not necessary for this procedure because it is noninvasive.
(C) obtaining the client's signature on an appropriate consent form following verbalized understanding of the procedure.
(D) giving an appropriate consent form to the client to be signed at a convenient time.

Physiological Integrity:
Pharmacological Therapies

Q–115

A physician's order indicates for a client to receive 0.45% sodium chloride at a continuous rate of 150 mL/hr. The nurse hangs a 1000 mL bag of the solution at 0800. When should the nurse expect a new bag will need to be hung?

(A) At around noon
(B) At around 2:30 PM
(C) At around 4 PM
(D) At around 6 PM

A–114

(C) Electrophysiologic study (EPS) is an invasive procedure that involves threading an electrode-tipped catheter through the femoral artery to the heart. The procedure is used to evaluate and treat cardiac arrhythmias that the client has experienced or is experiencing. Once the doctor has thoroughly explained an invasive procedure to a client, the task of obtaining consent may be delegated to the nurse. The nurse should have the client verbalize understanding of the procedure. If the client does not have any questions and shows an accurate understanding of the procedure, written consent in the form of a signature can be obtained on an appropriate consent form. Answer (C) is correct.

A–115

(B) At a rate of 150 mL/hr it will take 6.67 hours to infuse 1000 mL $\left(\frac{1000}{150} = 6.67\right)$. Therefore, the bag should be changed no later than shortly after 2:30 PM, which is $6\frac{1}{2}$ hours after the bag was first hung. Answer (B) is correct. The nurse should prevent letting all of the fluid infuse through the tubing prior to changing the bag to avoid air getting trapped in the tubing. At noon there should still be enough fluid in the bag for a couple more hours of infusion. A new bag needs to be hung before 4 PM or 6 PM to ensure continuous infusion according to the physician's order.

Physiological Integrity:
Physiological Adaptation

Q–116

The LPN/LVN is teaching a client regarding a newly diagnosed condition. The nurse states that the condition involves "uneven curvature of the cornea that leads to the inability of the retina to focus vision." Which of the following eye conditions does this statement represent?

(A) Astigmatism
(B) Glaucoma
(C) Myopia
(D) Cataracts

Physiological Integrity:
Physiological Adaptation

Q–117

The LPN/LVN is caring for an infant with hydrocephalus. Which of the following is most commonly the first sign of increased intracranial volume?

(A) Setting-sun sign
(B) Frontal bossing
(C) Cracked-pot sound
(D) Bulging fontanels

Answers

A–116

(A) This is an accurate description of what occurs with astigmatism, answer (A). Glaucoma is an increase in intraocular pressure caused by a disturbance in the circulation of aqueous fluid. Myopia is nearsightedness. Cataracts involve impaired vision or blindness caused by opacity of the lens or capsule of the eye.

A–117

(D) Various diseases can lead to hydrocephalus, which is caused by a disturbance of cerebrospinal fluid (CSF). CSF overfills beneath the skull bones, often causing the head to grow at an abnormal rate and intracranial volume and pressure to increase above normal. Bulging fontanels is usually the first sign of increased intracranial volume and pressure, answer (D). All answer choices are signs of hydrocephalus that occur later. Setting-sun sign is rotation of the eyes downward. Frontal bossing is frontal bone protrusion, which also causes the eyes to be depressed into the face. Cracked-pot sound is heard upon percussion of the skull. The skull bones are thin, and cranial sutures are separated.

Questions

Physiological Integrity:
Physiological Adaptation

Q–118

The LPN/LVN is developing the plan of care for an infant with myelomeningocele. Which of the following nursing diagnoses is least appropriate for this client?

(A) Risk for trauma related to delicate spinal lesion
(B) Risk for injury related to repeated exposure to latex products and potential for latex allergy development
(C) Risk for injury related to musculoskeletal impairment
(D) Risk for trauma related to impaired cerebrospinal fluid circulation

Safe and Effective Care Environment:
Safety and Infection Control

Q–119

While caring for a client with latex allergy, the LPN/LVN should be aware that clients with this type of allergy can have cross-reaction to which of the following foods? Select all that apply.

(A) Banana
(B) Walnut
(C) Avocado
(D) Kiwi
(E) Chestnut
(F) Citrus
(G) Coconut

A–118

(C) Myelomeningocele is a significant neural tube defect characterized by a hernial protrusion of a cyst from the spinal column. The delicate, saclike spinal lesion contains meninges, cerebrospinal fluid (CSF), and part of the spinal cord with its nerves. Due to exposure of spinal contents, these infants are highly susceptible to developing allergy to latex. CSF circulation is impaired as a cause of this herniation, which often leads to increased intracranial volume (hydrocephalus). This disorder is a neuromuscular disorder and does not involve the skeletal system. Answer (C) is the correct choice.

A–119

(A), **(C)**, **(D)**, and **(E)** are the correct answers. Latex allergy is a serious health hazard that can lead to anaphylaxis and death. Exaggerated precautions should be used with clients who are allergic to latex material. This includes knowing that contact with some foods can cause the same reaction as contact with latex in clients with this allergy. These foods include banana, avocado, kiwi, and chestnut. Walnut, citrus, and coconut have not been shown to cause cross-reactions in clients with a latex allergy.

Physiological Integrity:
Pharmacological Therapies

Q–120

Upon walking into the room in response to a client's call light, the LPN/LVN finds the client covered in hives and complaining of feeling very itchy. The physician prescribes a stat order for Benadryl 20 mg IM. The vial containing the medication reads 50 mg of Benadryl per mL. How much solution, in milliliters, should be administered?

(A) 0.2 mL
(B) 0.4 mL
(C) 1 mL
(D) 2 mL

Physiological Integrity:
Basic Care and Comfort

Q–121

Following a colonoscopy, the physician restricts the client to a clear liquid diet. Which of the following would be included as an allowed food for this diet?

(A) Gelatin
(B) Orange juice
(C) Ice cream
(D) Pudding

Answers

A–120

(B) Solve for x mL using the following ratio method.

$$\frac{50 \text{ mg}}{1 \text{ mL}} = \frac{20 \text{ mg}}{x \text{ mL}}$$

$$50x = 20$$

$$x = \frac{20}{50}$$

$$x = 0.4$$

The correct answer is (B).

A–121

(A) Clear liquids include any food or drink that liquefies at room temperature and is transparent. Gelatin, answer (A), is correct. Some fruit juices, such as grape and apple juice, are allowed. Orange juice can be too heavy and acidic for a client's digestive tract at this time. Other allowed foods and beverages include coffee, tea, fruit popsicles, clear carbonated beverages (i.e., ginger ale), and bouillon. Milk and dairy products can cause or intensify diarrhea and should be avoided until the gastrointestinal tract is better able to digest them.

Safe and Effective Care Environment:
Coordinated Care

Q–122

The LPN/LVN enters the client's room to obtain a signature on the consent form for a left inguinal hernia repair. The client states, "I hope I will be able to manage without part of my intestines." Which nursing action is appropriate at this time?

(A) Notify the physician.
(B) Shave the client's left groin.
(C) Say to the client, "We all have more intestines than we need anyway."
(D) Witness the client signing the form.

Physiological Integrity:
Pharmacological Therapies

Q–123

A physician order is written: Flagyl 250 mg po tid. Which of the following represents an appropriate administration schedule for this order?

(A) 0600, 1200, 1800, 0000
(B) 1000, 2200
(C) 0600, 1400, 2200
(D) 1000, 1600, 2200, 0400

A–122

(A) This statement indicates that the client does not understand the procedure that is to be performed. It is the physician's responsibility to explain the correct procedure and obtain consent. Without full knowledge of the invasive procedure to be done, the client's consent is not valid. The physician should be notified. Answer (A) is correct. Continuing with pre-operative procedures or having the client sign that he gives consent would not be appropriate without clarification of the situation. Answer (C) is not an appropriate response to the client's statement.

A–123

(C) Administration "tid" means the client should be given three of the prescribed doses of the medication a day, answer (C). All other choices either give more or less daily doses than prescribed. Administration schedules vary depending on the facility as long as the number of doses ordered by the physician is followed.

Safe and Effective Care Environment:
Coordinated Care

Q–124

The charge nurse would intervene if the LPN/LVN requested the unlicensed assistive personnel (UAP) to perform which tasks? Select all that apply.

(A) Assist a client who had a hip replacement three days ago with a bath.
(B) Change the dressing on the client who has a wound that is draining.
(C) Accompany the client who uses a walker to the bathroom.
(D) Perform vital signs on a client who will be discharged tomorrow.
(E) Ensure that a client finishes taking his medication.

Physiological Integrity:
Reduction of Risk Potential

Q–125

Diagnostic laboratory tests are used to monitor the function of organs in the body. Arrange the following tests according to the organs each is associated with, going from head to toe. (Use every answer choice provided.)

(A) Serum creatinine
(B) Troponin I
(C) PSA
(D) T_4

Answers

A-124

(B) and (E) The charge nurse would intervene if the LPN/LVN requested that the UAP perform a task that is beyond the scope of the UAP's practice. This would include asking a UAP to perform any type of dressing change on a client. It is the LPN/LVN's responsibility to ensure that a client completes taking the medication that has been administered. It is within the UAP's scope of practice to bathe a stable client, ambulate a client, and take vital signs.

A-125

The correct order is **(D)**, **(B)**, **(A)**, and **(C)**. The thyroid gland releases thyroxine (T_4) and triiodothyronine (T_3). Troponin I is a protein that is released into the blood following damage to the heart muscle. Elevated troponin I levels are looked for to indicate myocardial infarction (MI). Creatinine is a byproduct of muscle and protein metabolism that is excreted by the kidneys. Elevated serum creatinine indicates decreased kidney function. Prostate-specific antigen (PSA) is used to test for the existence of prostate cancer. The corresponding tests and organs are arranged in the following order from head to toe: T_4: thyroid gland; troponin I: heart; serum creatinine: kidneys; PSA: prostate.

Safe and Effective Care Environment:
Safety and Infection Control

Q–126

Which of the following actions by the LPN/LVN would demonstrate recognition of the most important method for controlling the spread of infection?

(A) The nurse applies clean gloves to change bed linens.
(B) The nurse applies sterile gloves during tracheostomy care.
(C) The nurse wears sterile gloves to empty a client's Foley bag.
(D) The nurse washes hands prior to and following contact with every client.

Safe and Effective Care Environment:
Coordinated Care

Q–127

A class of LPNs/LVNs is preparing for graduation. What document can LPNs/LVNs look to for the rules and regulations that define this license's scope of practice?

A–126

(D) Hand washing is the most important method in controlling spread of infection, answer (D). Hand washing breaks the chain of transmission of microorganisms. Wearing clean gloves and sterile gloves at appropriate times is also an important infection control method. Hand washing, however, has proven to be the most effective step in infection-control techniques. Sterile gloves are not necessary when emptying a Foley bag. Wearing clean gloves for this task is sufficient.

A–127

ANSWER: Nurse Practice Act
RATIONALE: The State Board of Nursing within each state is responsible for formulating the state's Nurse Practice Act, which documents the scope of practice for each type of nursing license (Registered Nurse, Licensed Practical Nurse/Licensed Vocational Nurse, Certified Nursing Assistant, etc.).

Safe and Effective Care Environment:
Coordinated Care

Q–128

An RN and two LPNs are caring for a group of clients. The RN is responsible for ensuring the physician's orders are completed. Which task would be inappropriate for the RN to delegate to the LPN?

(A) Inserting a Foley urinary catheter on a newly admitted but stable client
(B) Providing discharge instructions to a client
(C) Administering an IV push medication to a client in rapid ventricular rate atrial fibrillation (RVR A-fib)
(D) Removing a client's nasogastric tube on the third post-op day prior to discharge

Physiological Integrity:
Pharmacological Therapies

Q–129

The LPN/LVN is preparing to administer colchicine 0.5 mg po to a client. This nurse always prepares to explain the purpose for prescription of each medication prior to administering them. Which of the following is an appropriate reason for taking this medication?

(A) To treat rheumatoid arthritis
(B) To prevent recurrences of gouty arthritis
(C) To treat bronchitis
(D) To manage symptoms of congestive heart failure

A-128

(C) Although the regulations of state Nurse Practice Acts vary, the practical/vocational nurse should never be expected to care for an unstable client. A client in rapid ventricular rate atrial fibrillation (RVR A-fib)—an unpredictable cardiac arrhythmia—is not in a stable condition. The correct choice is answer (C). Most states also restrict LPNs/LVNs from administering medications via IV push. Depending on the allowed rate of administration, IV push medications go into the bloodstream in as little time as a few seconds.

A-129

(B) Used in larger doses to treat acute attacks and in smaller doses for prophylaxis, colchicine is an anti-gout agent. Colchicine is used to treat gouty arthritis, not rheumatoid arthritis. This medication is not used to treat bronchitis or for the management of congestive heart failure.

Physiological Integrity:
Pharmacological Therapies

Q–130

The physician writes a prescription for Benadryl to a client with severe hay fever symptoms. After looking over the medications that the client takes on a regular basis, which of the following should the LPN/LVN bring to the attention of the physician?

(A) Nardil
(B) Acetaminophen
(C) Digoxin
(D) Glucotrol

Safe and Effective Care Environment:
Safety and Infection Control

Q–131

A client receiving a blood transfusion becomes very anxious and dyspneic, and complains of chest tightness and back pain. The LPN/LVN recognizes that these could be signs of a transfusion reaction. Which of the following includes correct steps the nurse should take at this time?

(A) Slow the transfusion and notify the physician.
(B) Stop the transfusion, notify the physician and the blood bank.
(C) Activate the emergency response system, notify the physician, and obtain a urine sample.
(D) Distract the client to relieve anxiety and administer pain medication.

A–130

(A) Benadryl is an antihistamine used for treatment of allergies or hay fever. Drug-to-drug interactions include combined use with MAO inhibitors, such as Nardil. Acetaminophen is often used in conjunction with Benadryl to treat cold, flu, or allergy symptoms. Digoxin is an antiarrythmic used to increase cardiac output and slow rapid heart rates. There is no known interaction between Benadryl and Digoxin. Glucotrol is an oral hypoglycemic agent used for control of diabetes mellitus. There is no known interaction between Benadryl and Glucotrol.

A–131

(B) When a transfusion reaction is suspected, the following actions should be followed until the type and severity of the reaction is determined: stop the transfusion; maintain the IV line with normal saline infusion; carefully assess the client; notify the physician; notify the blood bank; return the blood product and all tubing to the blood bank for testing; and document the reaction according to policy. The nurse will need to collect a urine sample only if a hemolytic reaction or bacterial infection is suspected. Answer (B) is correct. Unless the client's condition is life threatening, it is not necessary to activate the emergency response system. Distracting the client is inappropriate during a transfusion reaction.

Safe and Effective Care Environment:
Safety and Infection Control

Q–132

Mrs. Thompson is receiving an infusion of fresh-frozen plasma. The client suddenly sits straight up in bed gasping for air. Her heart rate is elevated and crackles are heard at the base of the lungs upon auscultation. Which of the following conditions does this data suggest that Mrs. Thompson is experiencing?

(A) Allergic reaction to the blood product
(B) Acute hemolytic reaction to the blood product
(C) Pulmonary embolism
(D) Circulatory overload

Physiological Integrity:
Pharmacological Therapies

Q–133

A severely hyperglycemic client is placed on an insulin drip at 6 units/hr. The insulin is mixed in normal saline for administration. The solution contains 50 units per 100 mL. The LPN/LVN would calculate the rate of infusion to be how many mL/hr?

(A) 3 mL/hr
(B) 6 mL/hr
(C) 12 mL/hr
(D) 24 mL/hr

Answers

(D) Signs of circulatory overload include dyspnea, orthopnea, tachycardia, sudden anxiety, neck vein distention, crackles at the base of the lungs, and often the client experiences hypertension. Circulatory overload occurs when too much blood or blood product is infused too quickly. The symptoms exhibited are not typical of allergic reaction or acute hemolytic reaction to the blood product. Symptoms of pulmonary embolism include dyspnea, tachypnea, chest pain, fever, tachycardia, apprehension, cough, diaphoresis, hemoptysis, and syncope. These symptoms are similar to those the client is experiencing. However, the clinical situation and factors point to circulatory overload being the cause of the symptoms.

(C) Solve for x mL/hr using the following ratio method.

$$\frac{50 \text{ units}}{100 \text{ mL}} = \frac{6 \text{ units}}{x \text{ mL}}$$

$$50x = 600$$

$$x = \frac{600}{50}$$

$$x = 12 \text{ mL/hr}$$

The correct answer is (C).

Psychosocial Integrity

Q–134

The LPN/LVN is conversing with a resident at the long-term care facility. The resident asks, "What is the point of living when you can't do anything for yourself anymore?" Which of the following is a therapeutic response for the LPN/LVN to make?

(A) "You seem discouraged."
(B) "Things will get better. I promise."
(C) "Don't sound so depressed."
(D) "It's such a beautiful day today, isn't it?"

Physiological Integrity:
Basic Care and Comfort

Q–135

The LPN/LVN is inserting an indwelling catheter. The catheter was inserted into the urinary meatus, and urine is flowing through the catheter tubing. Prior to inflating the balloon, which of the following steps should be performed?

(A) Anchor the catheter to the client's thigh.
(B) Insert the catheter an additional 1 to 2 inches.
(C) Pull the catheter out 1 to 2 centimeters.
(D) Irrigate the bladder with 10 mL of sterile water.

Answers

(A) A therapeutic response by the nurse would be to direct this question back to the client, answer (A). This answer tells the client that the nurse sensed discouragement in the question and allows the client to explore whether or not this is what was meant by what was said. Answers (B), (C), and (D) are statements or questions that could hinder working through the client's thoughts and feelings. Answer (B) is offering unwarranted reassurance. Answer (C) is passing judgment. Answer (D) changes the topic and avoids the client's thoughts and feelings.

(B) Prior to inflating the balloon of an indwelling catheter, the catheter should be inserted one to two inches beyond the point at which urine is seen flowing. This prevents balloon inflation in the urethra, which could cause damage to the urinary structure. Answer (B) is correct. The catheter should be anchored after the balloon is properly inflated. If the catheter is pulled away from the bladder, the balloon would not be inflated inside the bladder. This could lead to balloon inflation in the urethra or removal of the catheter completely. Irrigation is not necessary during routine indwelling catheter insertion.

Safe and Effective Care Environment:
Coordinated Care

Q–136

Upon arrival at the hospital unit to begin the shift, the following four clients are assigned to the RN. The RN is working with an LPN and a CNA. Arrange the clients in order of priority to be seen by the RN.

(A) A confused elderly client with dementia who is continually trying to get out of bed
(B) A client ready for discharge after a cholecystectomy
(C) A client on continuous telemetry monitoring due to frequent episodes of ventricular tachycardia
(D) A client scheduled for an exploratory laparoscopy

Physiological Integrity:
Pharmacological Therapies

Q–137

A client who presented to the clinic with dysuria is diagnosed with a urinary tract infection. The physician prescribed phenazopyridine (Pyridium) to the client. Which of the following best describes the purpose of this medication?

(A) To kill the bacteria causing the infection
(B) To increase the acidity of the urine to prevent recurrent infection
(C) To take pressure off the bladder by increasing urinary output
(D) To relieve discomfort caused by the infection

A-136

The correct order is **(C)**, **(D)**, **(A)**, and **(B)**. The client who is on continuous telemetry monitoring and is experiencing frequent cardiac arrhythmias is the highest priority of these four clients. The RN should assume care of this client due to the critical nature of the condition. The RN can delegate preoperative care of the client scheduled for an exploratory laparoscopy to the LPN. The confused client can be monitored by the CNA until the RN is available. The client ready for discharge after a successful operation is of least priority.

A-137

(D) Phenazopyridine (Pyridium) is a urinary tract analgesic. Pyridium provides relief from pain, itching, and burning from the urinary tract infection as well as urinary urgency and frequency. The correct answer is (D). Pyridium is not an antimicrobial medication. Cranberry juice or acidic beverages are recommended to increase the acidity of urine which prevents bacterial growth and recurrent infection. Pyridium does not increase urinary output. The client is encouraged to increase fluid intake to dilute the urine.

Physiological Integrity:
Pharmacological Therapies

Q–138

The physician prescribes Pyridium to a client. The LPN/LVN reviews this medication with the client. The nurse should inform the client not to be alarmed by which of the following normal effects of this medication?

(A) High energy level
(B) Strange food cravings
(C) Orange-colored urine
(D) Increased olfactory sense

Physiological Integrity:
Basic Care and Comfort

Q–139

While monitoring a client's urinary output, the nurse is aware that an hourly output of less than which of the following amounts should be reported to the physician?

(A) 15 mL
(B) 30 mL
(C) 60 mL
(D) 100 mL

A-138

(C) A common side effect caused by the use of Pyridium is bright-orange urine. This is a normal effect. The client should be warned of this to avoid alarm when the effect is noticed. Pyridium does not cause a high energy level, strange food cravings, or an increased olfactory sense (sense of smell).

A-139

(B) Average urinary output at an hourly rate is 60 mL/hr. Urinary output less than 500 mL/day or 30 mL/hr is suggestive of renal insufficiency and impending renal failure. The correct answer is (B). The physician should be notified, and steps should be taken to promptly restore renal blood flow and urinary output to prevent renal complications and failure.

Physiological Integrity:
Basic Care and Comfort

Q–140

Mr. Franklin is a client on hemodialysis for end-stage renal disease (ESRD). The client receives hemodialysis through an arteriovenous fistula on his left forearm. Which of the following represents correct findings from assessment of the fistula's function?

(A) The nurse palpates a thrill and auscultates a bruit.
(B) The nurse palpates a bruit and auscultates a thrill.
(C) The nurse palpates a rush and auscultates a pulse.
(D) The nurse palpates a pulse and auscultates a rush.

Physiological Integrity:
Pharmacological Therapies

Q–141

The nurse is preparing to administer packed red blood cells (PRBCs) to a client. Which of the following fluids can be administered along with blood products using the same tubing and intravenous catheter site?

(A) 0.9% sodium chloride
(B) Dextrose 5% in water
(C) 0.45% sodium chloride
(D) Lactated Ringer's solution

Answers

(A) A thrill, a wavelike vibration indicating the flow of blood, should be palpable over the fistula, and a bruit, a swooshing sound indicating blood flow, should be heard upon auscultating the fistula. A *rush* is not a word used to describe a palpated or auscultated assessment. A pulse is not heard or felt at the fistula site.

(A) The only fluid solution that should ever be administered using any shared tubing or into the same intravenous catheter site with a blood product is 0.9% sodium chloride (normal saline). The correct answer is (A). Use of any other solution other than normal saline can cause the blood products to clot.

Q–142

The nurse has been caring for a client with dementia. What law may the nurse be violating by administering sedative medication to the client to keep the client quiet?

(A) Invasion of privacy
(B) Assault
(C) Battery
(D) False imprisonment

Q–143

The nurse is caring for a client who is near the end of life and begins to ask questions about different ways the client can leave items for his children after his death. When the nurse refers the client to seek expert legal advice, what role is the nurse demonstrating?

(A) Educator
(B) Communicator
(C) Advocate
(D) Case manager

A–142

(D) False imprisonment can be defined as using a chemical restraint (a sedative medication) to prevent a client from being loud or to get the client out of the nurse's way. Assault is threatening a client or saying something that makes a client feel threatened. Battery is touching a client in such a way that the client feels threatened. False imprisonment is holding a client against his/her will.

A–143

(C) The nurse as an advocate supports the client's right to make healthcare decisions and to prevent the client from harm when the client is unable to make decisions. The nurse as educator provides or reinforces teaching to the client. The nurse as communicator uses communication to address the needs of the client and to promote health and disease prevention. The nurse as case manager coordinates the care of the client.

Physiological Integrity:
Physiological Adaptation

Q–144

A client returns to the hospital unit after abdominal surgery. Which of the following assessment trends suggest that the client is going into shock?

(A) Increasing heart rate, decreasing blood pressure, decreasing urinary output
(B) Decreasing heart rate, increasing blood pressure, decreasing urinary output
(C) Increasing heart rate, increasing blood pressure, increasing urinary output
(D) Decreasing heart rate, decreasing blood pressure, increasing urinary output

---

Physiological Integrity:
Physiological Adaptation

Q–145

A nine-year-old boy is admitted to the pediatric unit with suspected meningitis. Which of the following is NOT commonly seen as a symptom of meningitis?

(A) Fever
(B) Tachycardia
(C) Stiff neck
(D) Photophobia

A–144

(A) Shock occurs when circulating blood volume decreases. Signs of decreasing circulating blood volume include an increase in heart rate, a decrease in blood pressure, and a decrease in urinary output. The heart pumps faster in an attempt to circulate the blood to the body parts. With a decrease in blood volume, stroke volume and pressure resistance against the pumping of the heart decreases, which leads to hypotension. Decreased blood volume leads to decreased renal perfusion of blood causing decreased urinary output. Answer (A) represents trends that occur as a client is going into shock.

A–145

(B) Meningitis is a serious condition involving inflammation of the membranes that surround the brain and spinal cord. Classic symptoms of meningitis include fever, headache, stiff neck, change in mental status, and photophobia (sensitivity to light). Some types of meningitis, such as acute bacterial meningitis, can cause seizures, shock, and death. Tachycardia is not a symptom caused by meningitis. The correct answer choice is (B).

Physiological Integrity:
Pharmacological Therapies

Q–146

Digoxin is a medication that requires maintaining a thera-peutic level in the blood. A digoxin level that is too high can be toxic. Which of the following are symptoms of digoxin toxicity? Select all choices that apply.

(A) Insomnia
(B) Nausea and vomiting
(C) Tachycardia
(D) Arrhythmias
(E) Yellow vision
(F) Hypertension
(G) Anorexia

Physiological Integrity:
Basic Care and Comfort

Q–147

Mrs. Stetson visits the clinic stating that she has not had a bowel movement in two days. The physician puts the client on a diet that is high in fiber. The LPN/LVN prepares dietary instruction on this type of diet. Which of the following in-cludes some of the best food choices?

(A) English muffin, chicken, canned carrots
(B) Pineapple, squash, cheddar cheese
(C) Corn flakes, potatoes, bagels
(D) Whole-grain bread, brown rice, oatmeal

A–146

(B), **(D)**, **(E)**, and **(G)** are the correct choices. Signs of digoxin toxicity include fatigue, arrhythmias, bradycardia, anorexia, nausea, vomiting, and yellow vision. Fatigue, not insomnia, is a sign of digoxin toxicity. Toxic levels of serum digoxin cause bradycardia as opposed to tachycardia. Digoxin is not known to affect blood pressure levels.

A–147

(D) Foods that are high in fiber include whole-grain breads, whole-grain hot or cold cereals, brown rice, beans, and popcorn. Foods prepared with refined flour such as regular English muffins, corn flakes, and plain bagels are not good sources of fiber. Dairy products can worsen symptoms of constipation. Fresh fruits and vegetables contain low to moderate amounts of fiber. Answer (D) includes the best food choices.

Physiological Integrity:
Basic Care and Comfort

Q–148

A client is diagnosed with acute cholecystitis and is scheduled for a cholecystectomy after the acute symptoms subside. In the meantime the client is instructed to avoid which types of foods?

(A) Cold foods
(B) Fibrous foods
(C) High-fat foods
(D) Foods high in sugar

Physiological Integrity:
Basic Care and Comfort

Q–149

The LPN/LVN is documenting in the nursing notes that the client has a decubitus ulcer that looks similar to a blister. In what stage is this decubitus ulcer?

(A) Stage I
(B) Stage II
(C) Stage III
(D) Stage IV

Answers

(C) Cholecystitis is inflammation of the gallbladder. The gall-bladder stores and concentrates bile, which functions in digestion of fats in food. Ingestion of high-fat foods stimulates the gallbladder, which in the presence of cholecystitis may bring on an acute episode. High-fat foods should be avoided, answer (C). The temperature of the food when it is ingested does not affect the digestion processes of the gallbladder. Gas-forming foods should be eaten only as tolerated, but fibrous foods do not need to be avoided with cholecystitis. Foods high in sugar are not con-traindicated with this condition.

(B) Stage II decubitus ulcers involve partial-thickness skin loss or blistering that can include epidermis and dermis layers of skin. Stage I decubitus ulcers are non-blanchable erythema of intact skin. Stage III decubitus ulcers involve full-thickness skin loss with damage to subcutaneous tissue. At this stage, the ulcer can be as deep as, but not through, the fascia layer. Stage IV decubitus ulcers involve full-thickness skin loss with tissue necrosis or damage to muscle, bone, or supporting structures.

Physiological Integrity:
Reduction of Risk Potential

Q–150

Which of the following would be the correct procedure to avoid contamination of a urine sample for urinalysis being obtained from a client's indwelling catheter?

(A) The nurse cleans the port on the drainage tubing with an alcohol wipe before withdrawing a sample using a syringe and needle.

(B) The nurse disconnects the drainage tubing from the indwelling catheter and uses a syringe to aspirate the sample through the catheter.

(C) The nurse keeps the collected sample in ice while transporting it to the laboratory.

(D) The nurse collects the sample from the drainage bag into a specimen container.

Safe and Effective Care Environment:
Coordinated Care

Q–151

A client is receiving a transfusion of packed red blood cells (PRBCs). The LPN/LVN knows that the most critical time to monitor a client receiving a blood transfusion is which of the following time intervals?

(A) 15 to 30 minutes after initiating the transfusion
(B) 1 to 2 hours after initiating the transfusion
(C) 15 minutes after the transfusion is completed
(D) 2 hours after the transfusion is completed

Answers

(A) Most indwelling catheters have a port on the tubing that allows samples to be withdrawn while preventing contamination. Wiping this port and withdrawing a sample using a syringe is correct procedure, answer (A). Sterile technique should be used anytime the indwelling catheter and the drainage tubing are disconnected as it is a closed system to maintain sterility of the urinary tract. Using a syringe to aspirate urine that has not left the bladder could be very harmful to the urinary tract. It is not necessary to refrigerate this sample prior to urinalysis testing. Other urine tests do require refrigeration. Sediment settles at the bottom of the drainage bag as the urine sits. Therefore, the urine in the drainage bag is not an appropriate sample of the client's urine composition.

(A) The majority of transfusion reactions occur within the first 15 to 30 minutes that the blood product is being transfused. Close monitoring of the client's vital signs is crucial at this time. The client should also be made aware of what they could experience during a transfusion reaction and to notify the nurse immediately if they experience any of these symptoms. Transfusion reactions typically occur within approximately the first 2 hours after the transfusion is begun.

Q–152

A severely anemic client is going to receive a blood transfusion of packed red blood cells (PRBCs). Prior to administering the blood product, the client must give consent. The LPN/LVN is reviewing the purpose of the blood transfusion along with potential symptoms the client could experience if a transfusion reaction occurs. Select all of the following that are signs or symptoms of a blood transfusion reaction.

(A) Urticaria
(B) Fever
(C) Chills
(D) Low back pain
(E) Dyspnea
(F) Nausea
(G) Hemoglobinuria
(H) Hypertension

A–152

(A) through (G) are all correct answers. Symptoms of an acute hemolytic reaction include fever, chills, low back pain, nausea, chest tightness, dyspnea, anxiety, hemoglobinuria (caused by RBC destruction and excretion by the kidneys), and hypotension. Answer (H) is the only incorrect answer. Symptoms of a febrile, nonhemolytic reaction include chills followed by a fever. Symptoms of an allergic reaction to a blood transfusion include urticaria (hives) and generalized itching. Hypertension may be present with fluid overload caused by a blood transfusion.

Q–153

Mr. Thompson undergoes diagnostic testing that confirms existence of a deep vein thrombosis (DVT) in his left leg. The client is placed on anticoagulant therapy with Lovenox (low-molecular weight heparin) injections and oral Coumadin. Mr. Thompson asks the nurse why he has to take two medications to treat this condition. Which of the following is an appropriate response to this question by the LPN/LVN?

(A) "The combined use helps break up the clot faster."
(B) "The Lovenox is a temporary treatment until the Coumadin becomes therapeutic."
(C) "Lovenox breaks down the already existent clot while Coumadin prevents more clots from forming."
(D) "Coumadin prevents further clot formation while Lovenox prevents the clot in your leg from traveling through the bloodstream to the lungs."

(B) Warfarin (Coumadin) is the drug of choice for long-term anticoagulation therapy because it can be taken orally. However, Coumadin takes 48 to 72 hours to reach a therapeutic level in the blood stream. To obtain the immediate effects of anticoagulation, a form of heparin is used temporarily, either by injection or intravenous administration. Heparin becomes therapeutic in the bloodstream within a few hours. Anticoagulation agents do not break up clots that are already existent or prevent existent clots from moving through the blood stream. These medications are used to prevent further clot formation. Answer (B) is correct.

Physiological Integrity:
Pharmacological Therapies

Q–154

A client with recurrent DVTs is placed on anticoagulation therapy. Which of the following values indicates that warfarin (Coumadin) is at a therapeutic level for anticoagulation?

(A) International normalized ratio (INR) of 1.6
(B) Prothrombin time (PT) of 13 seconds
(C) Activated partial thromboblastin time (APTT) of 36 seconds
(D) International normalized ratio (INR) of 2.4

Physiological Integrity:
Pharmacological Therapies

Q–155

A client is receiving aminophylline 500 mg IV mixed in 500 mL over 12 hours. How much medication does the client receive in 1 hr using this rate?

(A) 500 mg/hr
(B) 60 mg/hr
(C) 42 mg/hr
(D) 0.7 mg/hr

Answers

(**D**) Prothrombin time (PT) and international normalized ratio (INR) are used to monitor response to oral anticoagulation therapy, such as Coumadin therapy. The therapeutic range for PT while on anticoagulation therapy is 15 to 28 seconds. The therapeutic range for INR while on anticoagulation therapy to treat DVTs is 2.0 to 3.0. Answer (D) is correct. APTT is used to monitor response to heparin therapy. Desirable values for APTT while on heparin therapy are determined by the physician.

(**C**) 500 mg/500 mL = 1 mg/1 mL. To calculate the number of mL given over one hour, divide the total number of mL of solution by the number of hours used to infuse the solution. 500 mL/12 hours = 41.666 or 42 mL = 42 mg. The correct answer is (C).

Q–156

Mrs. Springer is pregnant in her 34th week of gestation. During a routine visit, the physician orders a biophysical profile. Select all of the following variables that are assessed by this exam.

(A) Fetal breathing movement
(B) Fetal heart rate (FHR) reactivity
(C) Amniotic fluid volume
(D) Fetal tone
(E) Fetal arrhythmias
(F) Placental function

Q–157

A biophysical profile is a diagnostic procedure that combines which of the following?

(A) Non-stress test and sonogram
(B) Contraction stress test and sonogram
(C) Amniocentesis and contraction stress test
(D) Amniocentesis and non-stress test

A–156

(A), **(B)**, **(C)**, and **(D)** are correct answers. A biophysical profile is used to determine the risk of intrauterine compromise to the fetus by assessing five fetal biophysical variables. These variables are breathing movement, body movement, tone, amniotic fluid volume, and fetal heart rate (FHR) reactivity. Fetal echocardiography is used to assess cardiac structures and allow for treatment of fetal arrhythmias. Placental function is examined using a couple of different tests, Doppler velocimetry and contraction stress tests.

A–157

(A) A biophysical profile uses sonography to evaluate fetal breathing movement, fetal body movement, fetal tone, and amniotic fluid volume. A non-stress test is performed to evaluate fetal heart rate (FHR) reactivity. A score of 0 to 2 is given to each of the 5 factors, with a maximum score of 10. A score ranging from 8 to 10, with normal amniotic fluid volume, is considered acceptable and intervention is unnecessary. The contraction stress test evaluates respiratory function of the placenta. Amniocentesis is a procedure that involves the use of a needle and syringe to withdraw a sample of amniotic fluid for genetic, biochemical, or other testing and/or for correction of hydramnios (condition of too much amniotic fluid in the uterus).

Q–158

The physician has ordered "tap-water enemas until clear" for an adult client. The LPN/LVN has prepared the client and lubricated the tip of the rectal tube. How far should the nurse insert the rectal tube?

(A) 2.5 to 3.75 cm
(B) 5 to 7.5 cm
(C) 7 to 10 cm
(D) approximately 12 cm

Q–159

The LPN/LVN is inserting a rectal tube for administration of a tap-water enema. Which of the following is a correct action in this procedure?

(A) The client should assume a right lateral position to facilitate flow of solution by gravity into the sigmoid and descending colon.
(B) The solution container should be held at 20 in. above the rectum.
(C) To follow the direction of the rectum, the rectal tube should be pointed toward the spine upon insertion.
(D) To follow the direction of the rectum, the rectal tube should be pointed toward the umbilicus upon insertion.

A–158

(C) The tip of the catheter needs to go beyond the anal sphincter, which in an adult is located approximately 2.5 to 5 cm into the rectum beyond the anus. Therefore, to ensure the tip is past this point, it should be inserted 7 to 10 cm into the rectum. The rectal tube should be inserted 5 to 7.5 cm for a child and 2.5 to 3.75 cm for an infant. Twelve centimeters is farther than necessary.

A–159

(D) The rectal tube should be inserted to follow the direction of the rectum. This involves pointing the tube toward the umbilicus when inserting. Pointing the rectal tube toward the spine when inserting could cause pain and injury to the client. The client should be in a left lateral position to facilitate flow of solution by gravity into the sigmoid and descending colon. The higher the solution container is held above the rectum, the faster the flow and the greater the pressure in the rectum. For a normal enema, the container should be held no higher than 30 cm (or 12 in.) above the rectum. For a high enema, where the solution must go farther into the intestines, the container should be held no higher than 45 cm (or 18 in.) above the rectum.

Physiological Integrity:
Pharmacological Therapies

Q–160

Mr. Spencer is a client on chemotherapy for throat cancer. The client begins experiencing severe nausea. Of the following prn medications that this client is prescribed, which would the LPN/LVN administer for relief of this symptom?

(A) Alprazolam
(B) Promethazine
(C) Loperamide
(D) Meperidine

Physiological Integrity:
Basic Care and Comfort

Q–161

A client with actively bleeding esophageal varices is being admitted to the unit. Which type of nasogastric tube will most likely be inserted as a part of the treatment for this condition?

(A) Levin
(B) Gastric sump
(C) Moss
(D) Sangstaken-Blakemore

A-160

(B) Promethazine (or Phenergan) is an antiemetic used to diminish nausea and/or vomiting, answer (B). Alprazolam (or Xanax) is an antianxiety agent. Loperamide (or Imodium) is an antidiarrheal medication. Meperidine (or Demerol) is an opioid analgesic to treat pain.

A-161

(D) Esophageal varices are dilated veins that are most commonly found in the lower esophagus. These veins bleed or sometimes burst, leading to severe blood loss. Sangstaken-Blakemore tubes are used to treat esophageal varices. This type of tube inflates to compress the esophageal wall and provide pressure to the bleeding sites. Levin tubes and Gastric sump tubes are short nasogastric tubes, which are most commonly used to remove gas and fluid from the upper GI tract. These tubes are sometimes used for gastric feeding as well. Moss tubes are most commonly used for postoperative feeding and gastric decompression.

Health Promotion and Maintenance

Q–162

The LPN/LVN is teaching a client recently diagnosed with Ménière's disease about ways to reduce the presence and severity of symptoms during an acute episode. Which of the following is an inappropriate intervention for the nurse to teach the client?

(A) Relax in a comfortable chair and watch television to improve relaxation during an exacerbation.
(B) Decrease caffeine consumption.
(C) Follow a low-sodium diet (2000 mg/day).
(D) Antihistamines can help lessen symptoms.

Physiological Integrity:

Basic Care and Comfort

Q–163

During a routine physical exam at the clinic, a client is asked to provide a urine sample for urinalysis. Which of the following would NOT be included in the results of this test?

(A) Presence of glucose in the urine
(B) Urine clarity and odor
(C) Types of bacteria in the urine
(D) Measurement of urine pH

Answers

A–162

(A) Ménière's disease is a condition caused by fluid build-up in the inner ear. Symptoms include vertigo, progressive deafness, tinnitus, and a feeling of fullness in the ears. Appropriate interventions for reducing symptoms of Ménière's disease include: a low sodium diet to decrease fluid retention; avoiding caffeine, nicotine, and alcohol, which cause vasoconstriction; use of prescribed medications such as antihistamines, antiemetics, and Antivert to reduce symptoms such as nausea and vertigo; and reducing surrounding stimuli. Answer (A) is the correct answer choice. Television involves visual and audible stimuli, which can exacerbate symptoms of Ménière's disease.

A–163

(C) A urinalysis includes: observation of urine color, clarity, and odor; measurement of urine pH and specific gravity; detection of protein, glucose, and ketone in the urine; and microscopic examination of the urine sediment to detect red blood cells, white blood cells, casts, crystals, pus, and bacteria. Types of bacteria in the urine are not tested with a basic urinalysis, making (C) the correct answer. There should not be bacteria in the urine. If bacteria is found, a culture of the urine sample will be performed to identify the bacterial types.

Physiological Integrity:
Basic Care and Comfort

Q–164

A 17-year-old female presents to the clinic with a complaint of persistent fatigue. The client is diagnosed with iron deficiency anemia. It is discovered during the medical history that the client has been skipping meals and cutting back on certain foods in order to lose weight. Which of the following food groups, when removed from the diet would contribute the most to iron deficiency anemia?

(A) Fruits
(B) Meats
(C) Vegetables
(D) Dairy

Physiological Integrity:
Pharmacological Therapies

Q–165

The physician prescribes the following for a client: Regular insulin 15 units mixed with NPH insulin 20 units subcutaneously at 7 AM and 7 PM. The LPN/LVN preparing the medication for administration draws up the medication into the same syringe. Arrange the following answer choices into the order that is correct for mixing these medications from separate vials.

(A) Inject air into the vial of regular insulin.
(B) Draw 15 units of medication from the vial of regular insulin.
(C) Inject air into the vial of NPH insulin.
(D) Draw 20 units of medication from the vial of NPH insulin.

Answers

A-164

(B) All forms of meat and fish are good sources of iron. There are other good sources of iron such as some kinds of beans, iron-fortified cereal, whole grains, and leafy green vegetables. However, omission of the meat food group from the diet would cause the largest deficiency of dietary iron, which would contribute greatly to iron deficiency anemia. The correct answer is (B). Some vegetables do provide a good source of iron, but iron is not absorbed as well from vegetables as from other sources. Fruits and dairy products are not good sources of iron.

A-165

The correct order is **(C)**, **(A)**, **(B)**, and **(D)**. To prevent inserting regular (fast-acting) insulin into the vial of NPH (intermediate-acting) insulin, the LPN/LVN should use the following steps for mixing these medications in a syringe: draw up the amount of air equivalent to the total number of units to be administered; inject the amount of air equivalent to the ordered number of NPH units into the NPH vial; withdraw the needle; inject the remaining air into the regular insulin vial; withdraw the ordered amount of regular insulin; withdraw the needle; and withdraw the ordered amount of NPH insulin.

Safe and Effective Care Environment:
Safety and Infection Control

Q–166

A client in respiratory distress is receiving oxygen therapy through a non-rebreather mask set at 12 liters of oxygen per minute to maintain a satisfactory respiratory condition. The LPN/LVN knows that a non-rebreather mask set at 12 liters of oxygen per minute is providing approximately which of the following concentrations of oxygen?

(A) 50% to 60%
(B) 60% to 70%
(C) 70% to 80%
(D) 80% to 100%

Physiological Integrity:
Reduction of Risk Potential

Q–167

The LPN/LVN knows that a client on a non-rebreather mask is obtaining a high concentration of oxygen, which can lead to oxygen toxicity after prolonged use. Select all of the following signs and symptoms that would suggest the client is experiencing oxygen toxicity.

(A) Nausea
(B) Dyspnea
(C) Substernal chest pain
(D) Fatigue
(E) Confusion
(F) Numbness in the legs and hands

Answers

(D) A non-rebreather mask set at 12 liters of oxygen per minute is delivering 80% to 100% O_2. The suggested flow rate for a non-rebreather mask is 12 L/min of O_2. A partial rebreather mask set at the suggested flow rate of 8 to 11 L/min of O_2 would be delivering between 50% and 75% O_2. A simple mask set at the suggested flow rate of 6 to 8 L/min O_2 would be delivering between 40% and 60% O_2. These are the common methods of delivering O_2 saturations greater than 50%.

Answers **(B)**, **(C)**, **(D)**, and **(F)** are all signs and symptoms of oxygen toxicity. Oxygen toxicity can occur when a concentration of greater than 50% of O_2 is administered for longer than 48 hours. Signs and symptoms of oxygen toxicity include substernal distress, paresthesias (numbness and tingling of the extremities), dyspnea, restlessness, fatigue, malaise, progressive respiratory difficulty, hypoventilation, and infiltration of fluid into the alveoli. Confusion and nausea are not caused by oxygen toxicity.

Psychosocial Integrity

Q–168

Concerned parents place an EMS call for their 15-year-old son after finding him abusing cocaine in his room. The boy is brought to the emergency room. Select all of the following that are clinical manifestations of cocaine overdose.

(A) Hypotension
(B) Tachycardia
(C) Seizures
(D) Dysrhythmias
(E) High fever
(F) Nausea and vomiting
(G) Lethargy

Safe and Effective Care Environment:
Safety and Infection Control

Q–169

The LPN/LVN at the clinic answers a phone call. In a state of panic, the woman's voice on the line explains to the nurse that her husband started choking while eating a piece of steak. Which of the following questions should the LPN/LVN ask first?

(A) "Is your husband coughing?"
(B) "Is there anyone there besides you and your husband?"
(C) "Is your husband standing or sitting?"
(D) "Is your husband able to swallow?"

(B), **(C)**, **(D)**, and **(E)** are correct answers. Cocaine, a CNS stimulant, can cause the following symptoms: tachycardia, hypertension, hyperpyrexia (high fevers), seizures, and ventricular dysrhythmias. Other manifestations associated with cocaine use are euphoria, anxiety, sadness, insomnia, sexual indifference, hallucinations with delusions, psychosis, extreme paranoia, and hypervigilance. Cocaine overdose would cause hypertension as opposed to hypotension. Nausea and vomiting are withdrawal symptoms of cocaine but are not seen in situations of overdose. Cocaine abuse would cause insomnia, not lethargy.

(A) The most important piece of information to find out is if the airway is completely or partially obstructed. If the choking victim is able to move any air through the airway, he will be able to cough and expel the object without assistance. Answer (A) is correct. Helping the choking victim during a partial obstruction could cause more harm than it would help. If the obstruction progresses to a complete obstruction, a second person could then intervene. The victim's position, whether or not there is anyone else there, and the ability of the victim to swallow is not information that is necessary at this time.

Q–170

The physician writes an order as follows: piperacillin 2 g IM q 4 hours. The LPN/LVN reconstitutes the medication in a vial using the instructions on the label. The label indicates to add 4 mL of sterile water to the vial, which contains 2 g of piperacillin, to yield 1 g piperacillin per 2.5 mL solution. How much solution should the LPN/LVN draw into the syringe for administration?

(A) 2.5 mL
(B) 3 mL
(C) 4 mL
(D) 5 mL

Q–171

The LPN/LVN is suctioning the airway of an intubated client using a closed suction system. The nurse should apply suction by occluding the vent on the suction catheter at which of the following times?

(A) Before inserting the suction catheter into the cannula of the tracheostomy
(B) Once the tip of the suction catheter is no longer visible
(C) While withdrawing the suction catheter
(D) When the client begins gagging

Answers

(D) Solve for x mL using the following ratio method.

$$\frac{1 \text{ g}}{2.5 \text{ mL}} = \frac{2 \text{ g}}{x \text{ mL}}$$

$$1x = 5$$

$$x = 5$$

The correct answer is (D).

(C) Suction should be applied only after full insertion of the suction catheter, during withdrawal, to decrease the amount of oxygen that is pulled from the client's airway. Applying suction prior to insertion of the catheter or just inside the tracheostomy increases the potential for hypoxemia by increasing the amount of time that oxygenated air is removed from the airway. Gagging does not indicate the proper time to initiate suction.

Physiological Integrity:
Reduction of Risk Potential

Q–172

The LPN/LVN is performing tracheostomy care for a client. While suctioning the tube, the nurse should apply suction for no longer than

(A) 5 seconds
(B) 10 seconds
(C) 15 seconds
(D) 20 seconds

Physiological Integrity:
Basic Care and Comfort

Q–173

Mrs. Allen is a client on the medical floor with severe emphysema. The LPN/LVN is assisting the client with morning care. A client with emphysema commonly exhibits which of the following?

(A) Pigeon chest
(B) Kyphoscoliosis
(C) Barrel-shaped chest
(D) Funnel-shaped chest

A–172

(B) Applying suction for longer than 10 seconds can cause hypoxemia by pulling oxygenated air from the client's airway. The correct answer is (B). Suctioning for too little time may not effectively clear the airway. The minimum amount of time that suctioning is applied is usually 5 seconds. Holding suction for 15 or 20 seconds could lead to severe hypoxemia.

A–173

(C) Caused by over inflation of the lungs when air becomes trapped in the alveoli, clients with emphysema commonly have a chest that is said to be "barrel-shaped." Pigeon chest is caused by displacement of the sternum that may occur from rickets or Marfan syndrome. Kyphoscoliosis is an elevation of the scapula resulting in an S-shaped spine that can be caused by osteoporosis or other skeletal malformations. Funnel-shaped chest is caused by a depression of the sternum and may occur with rickets or Marfan syndrome.

Physiological Integrity:
Reduction of Risk Potential

Q–174

A client is experiencing severe dyspnea during an asthma attack. Which of the following adventitious sounds is characteristic of the onset of asthma symptoms?

(A) Low-pitched wheezing on expiration
(B) Crackles in early inspiration
(C) Pleural friction rub
(D) High-pitched wheezing on inspiration and expiration

Physiological Integrity:
Pharmacological Therapies

Q–175

The LPN/LVN is preparing to administer theophylline (Theobid) intravenously to a client. Which of the following is NOT a common side effect caused by use of this medication?

(A) Bradycardia
(B) Seizures
(C) Nausea and vomiting
(D) Anxiety

A–174

(**D**) Asthma is a pulmonary disorder caused by inflammation and narrowing of the air passages. High-pitched wheezing that occurs on inspiration and/or expiration is characteristic of asthma. Answer (D) is correct. Low-pitched wheezing heard on expiration usually suggests secretions in the airway, indicating the client needs to cough. Crackles in early inspiration are characteristic of COPD, pneumonia, and bronchitis. Pleural friction rub indicates loss of pleural fluid and inflammation of pleural tissues.

A–175

(**A**) Theophylline (Theobid) is a bronchodilator used for long-term control of asthma or COPD symptoms. Common side effects include seizures, anxiety, arrhythmias, tachycardia, and nausea and vomiting. The correct answer choice is (A). Theophylline (Theobid) causes tachycardia as opposed to bradycardia.

Safe and Effective Care Environment:
Safety and Infection Control

Q–176

A community health nurse is providing education to high school students regarding the human immunodeficiency virus (HIV). During discussion on preventing transmission of the disease, the nurse would be correct in pointing out that

(A) it is very unlikely for a woman to become infected by unprotected intercourse with an HIV positive man.

(B) use of oral contraceptives increases a woman's susceptibility to HIV.

(C) use of spermicides with nonoxyl 9 increases susceptibility to HIV for both men and women.

(D) as long as condoms are used appropriately, transmission of the HIV infection will not occur during intercourse.

Physiological Integrity:
Reduction of Risk Potential

Q–177

Which of the following is a laboratory test used to diagnose human immunodeficiency virus (HIV)?

(A) Western blot antibody test

(B) Quantitative plasma culture

(C) Percentage of CD4+ cells

(D) CD4 cell function test

Answers

(B) Elevated estrogen levels in women who use oral contraceptives have been found to increase the likelihood for becoming infected with human immunodeficiency virus (HIV) as a result of sexual relations with HIV positive partners. It is very likely for transmission of the HIV infection to occur during unprotected sex. It is more likely for women to contract the disease during intercourse than for men. Spermicides with nonoxyl 9 used during intercourse decrease HIV transmission. The only 100% effective method for preventing sexual transmission of HIV is abstinence.

(A) Tests used for diagnosis of human immunodeficiency virus (HIV) look for antibodies to the virus in a client's body. Four tests are used for this purpose: enzyme-linked immunosolvent assay (ELISA), western blot antibody test, indirect immuno-fluorescence assay (IFA), and radioimmunoprecipitation assay (RIPA). Answer (A) is correct. Quantitative plasma culture is a test used to track the progression of the disease and response to treatment. Testing for the percentage of CD4+ cells present and CD4 cell function is used to determine a client's immune status.

Q–178

A client is hospitalized due to complications of acquired immunodeficiency syndrome (AIDS). The wife of the client asks the nurse to explain the difference between AIDS and human immunodeficiency virus (HIV). Of the following, which contains the most accurate information?

(A) "AIDS requires medical treatment and HIV does not."
(B) "HIV is a latent form of the AIDS virus."
(C) "AIDS is a condition caused by infection with HIV."
(D) "Once infected with HIV, a person becomes more susceptible to the AIDS virus."

Q–179

A 28-year-old HIV positive female client is diagnosed with AIDS after testing is conducted to measure her CD4+ helper T-cell count. Of the following CD4+ helper T-cell count results, which indicates AIDS diagnosis for a client who is HIV positive?

(A) 200 cells/mm^3
(B) 184 cells/mm^3
(C) 300 cells/mm^3
(D) 215 cells/mm^3

Answers

(C) Acquired immunodeficiency syndrome (AIDS) is the state of depressed immunity that occurs as a result of human immunodeficiency virus (HIV) infection. Answer (C) is correct. For clients to be diagnosed with AIDS, they must be infected with HIV and have signs of low immune levels according to serum tests or an opportunistic infection or an AIDS-defining malignancy. A combination of any or all of these symptoms may be present in AIDS. Both AIDS and HIV require medical treatment. HIV is the virus that may lead to AIDS. It is not a latent form of AIDS. AIDS is not a virus.

(B) A count of less than 200 CD4+ helper T-cells/mm^3 is diagnostic of AIDS in clients that are HIV positive. Asymptomatic HIV positive clients with cell counts of 200 cells/mm^3 or higher are not considered to have AIDS. Answers (A), (C), and (D) are cell counts at or above this level.

Safe and Effective Care Environment:
Safety and Infection Control

Q–180

Opportunistic infections occur as a result of immune system malfunction. The most common infection found in people with AIDS is

(A) Kaposi's sarcoma
(B) *Mycobacterium avium* complex
(C) *Clostridium difficile* diarrhea
(D) *Pneumocystis jiroveci* pneumonia

Safe and Effective Care Environment:
Coordinated Care

Q–181

The nurse is caring for a woman who has just given birth and is considering relinquishing the child for adoption. What statement by the nurse may assist this client in this decision?

(A) "I think whatever you decide will work out."
(B) "Do you have enough money to support this child?"
(C) "Can you describe to me the options you have available to you?"
(D) "Adoption will give your child many opportunities unavailable to you now."

Answers

A–180

(D) All of the choices are common diseases seen in clients with AIDS, but answer (D), *Pneumocystis jiroveci* pneumonia, is the most common infection. This is one of the first opportunistic infections identified to be a disease associated with AIDS. Kaposi's sarcoma is the most common HIV-related malignancy. *Mycobacterium avium* complex is a group of bacteria that causes infection of the respiratory or gastrointestinal (GI) tracts. *Clostridium difficile* diarrhea is also a commonly seen GI tract infection in AIDS clients.

A–181

(C) The nurse can help clients who are involved in an ethical decision to clarify their values. When the nurse asks the client to describe the options available in this situation, it assists the client to examine all of the options and to explore options that may not seem feasible. The nurse does not assist with values clarification by saying that any decision will be fine or that the client cannot provide adequately for the child.

Safe and Effective Care Environment:
Safety and Infection Control

Q–182

While attending a seminar on the human immunodeficiency virus (HIV) and acquired immunodeficiency syndrome (AIDS), a student nurse identifies modes for transmission of HIV. Of the following actions, which could likely result in transmission of HIV? (Select all choices that apply.)

(A) Intravenous needle sharing with an infected individual
(B) Touching hands to mouth after shaking hands with an infected individual
(C) Blood products acquired from an infected individual used for transfusion in another individual
(D) Sharing drinking straws with an infected individual
(E) In-utero transfer from mother to fetus
(F) Transfer via breast milk from mother to newborn
(G) Engaging in oral sex with an infected individual

Physiological Integrity:
Reduction of Risk Potential

Q–183

A client with a decubitus ulcer on his coccyx has wet-to-dry dressings changed daily. An appropriate response from the LPN/LVN when the client asks about the purpose of this type of dressing would be:

(A) "This dressing helps protect the wound."
(B) "This dressing absorbs drainage from the wound."
(C) "This dressing aids in the removal of dead tissue from the wound."
(D) "This dressing cleans the wound and prevents infection."

Answers

(A), (C), (E), (F), and (G) are correct. Transmission of human immunodeficiency virus (HIV) occurs by way of body fluids containing the actual virus or CD4+ lymphocytes from an infected individual. Body fluids containing these cells include serum, seminal fluid, vaginal secretions, amniotic fluid, and breast milk. Anytime contact occurs between these fluids from an infected individual and another person, transmission is possible. Likelihood of transmission increases as contaminated body fluids come into contact with areas of the body that access the circulatory system more readily. The virus is not transmitted by shaking hands. Transmission is not likely to occur through exchange of saliva as in sharing a drinking straw.

(C) Wet-to-dry dressings are used for debridement, which is removal of necrotic (dead) tissue. The necrotic tissue is softened by the dressing when it is wet, and as the dressing dries the tissue sticks to the dressing. When the dressing is removed, the necrotic tissue is pulled from the wound. A dry-to-dry dressing is used to protect and absorb drainage from wounds. A wet-to-wet dressing keeps the wound continually bathed and helps prevent infection.

Physiological Integrity:

Basic Care and Comfort

Q-184

The physician orders urinary catheterization to obtain a urine sample from a female client. In preparation for the procedure, the nurse should place the client in the

(A) dorsal recumbent position
(B) supine position
(C) lithotomy position
(D) Sim's position

Physiological Integrity:

Reduction of Risk Potential

Q-185

The nurse obtains arterial blood gas results from a client with chronic emphysema. Which of the following acid-base disturbances is most commonly caused by chronic emphysema?

(A) Metabolic acidosis
(B) Metabolic alkalosis
(C) Respiratory acidosis
(D) Respiratory alkalosis

Answers

(A) For urinary catheterization the best position for a female would be dorsal recumbent. This involves lying on the back with the knees flexed and the soles of the feet placed flat on the lying surface. Supine position involves lying flat on a surface with both legs extended. This position is used for assessment of the head, neck, chest, and abdomen. Lithotomy position is a back-lying position with feet supported in stirrups. This is used during female pelvic examination. Sim's position is a side-lying position that is used to examine the rectum.

(C) Emphysema is a type of chronic obstructive pulmonary disease in which the air spaces in the lungs are distended due to trapping of air. This air trapping causes carbon dioxide that would normally be exhaled to be retained in the body and travel from the lungs to the pulmonary circulation. Respiratory acidosis is always a result of inadequate disposal of CO_2 during respiration. Metabolic acidosis is often seen with renal failure. Metabolic alkalosis can be caused by vomiting, gastric suctioning, or other conditions that involve loss of gastric contents. Respiratory alkalosis is a result of hyperventilation.

Physiological Integrity:
Basic Care and Comfort

Q–186

A client with chronic obstructive pulmonary disease (COPD) develops shortness of breath (SOB). The LPN/LVN knows that for clients with COPD, oxygen supplementation

(A) should always be administered with a mask.
(B) is adjusted according to client's comfort.
(C) should be administered and adjusted with extreme caution.
(D) is always provided at 6 liters/minute by way of a nasal cannula.

Physiological Integrity:
Pharmacological Therapies

Q–187

A client develops "dumping syndrome" following a vagotomy. Select all of the following that are used for the medical management of this condition.

(A) Antispasmodics
(B) Dietary supplementation of triglycerides
(C) Imodium
(D) Octreotide (Sandostatin)
(E) NSAIDs
(F) Corticosteroidal therapy

Answers

A-186

(C) Respiratory drive in a healthy person is stimulated by high levels of $PaCO_2$ that need to be exhaled. In clients with COPD, $PaCO_2$ levels are often chronically high, which suppresses this response to CO_2 and causes respirations to be stimulated by a hypoxic drive. This means that low levels of oxygen in the body stimulate inspiration. If oxygen is administered at too high of a rate to persons with this condition, respirations may cease due to lack of drive. There is not a standard rate or device used for administering oxygen to clients with any disease or condition. Oxygen supplementation is not adjusted primarily for client comfort but for respiratory need.

A-187

(A), **(B)**, and **(D)** are correct. "Dumping syndrome" is a condition that results from rapid movement of foods through the gastrointestinal (GI) tract following gastric surgery. Treatment for "dumping syndrome" includes use of any or all of the following: antispasmodics to delay gastric emptying; octreotide (Sandostatin), an anti-diarrheal that slows gastric emptying; dietary monitoring; dietary supplementation of triglycerides; vitamin B_{12}; and iron supplementation by injections (when dietary intake shows to be inadequate). Use of Imodium, an anti-diarrheal, may lead to chronic dependence. NSAIDs and corticosteroids are used to treat inflammatory conditions, and both of these medications are irritants to the GI tract mucosa.

Safe and Effective Care Environment:
Safety and Infection Control

Q–188

A client has an allergy to shellfish. This information is important to provide to all medical staff because it contraindicates diagnostic testing with the use of what substance?

Physiological Integrity:
Pharmacological Therapies

Q–189

A client complains of ringing in the ears. The nurse reviews the client's daily medications because this may be a sign of toxic levels of

(A) Tylenol
(B) aspirin
(C) Vistaril
(D) Claritin

A–188

ANSWER: Iodine

RATIONALE: Many diagnostic tests use dyes that contain iodine. Clients with an allergy to shellfish are known to have sensitivity to iodine as well. This information is important for the nurse, physician, and any technicians involved in diagnostic procedures. Alternative testing methods are usually available.

A–189

(B) Tinnitus, or ringing in the ears, is an early sign of toxicity that can occur from daily use of high dosages of aspirin. Tinnitus is a persistent ringing, buzzing, whistling, or other type of sound that is not caused by external stimuli. Tinnitus is not an effect known to be caused by Tylenol. Vistaril and Claritin are antihistamines. These medications are also not known to cause tinnitus.

Q–190

A client diagnosed with acromegaly visits the health clinic. The LPN/LVN would expect to discover which of the following manifestations with assessment of this client?

(A) Deep voice
(B) Small hands and feet
(C) Hearing loss
(D) Elephantiasis

Q–191

A client with a rectal tumor undergoes an abdominal perineal resection with placement of a permanent sigmoid colostomy. Instruction provided by the LPN/LVN regarding the function and care of the colostomy includes which of the following?

(A) "It will take 3 to 6 days for the colostomy to begin functioning."
(B) "An abrasive cleanser is used to clean the stoma."
(C) "Foods to avoid with a colostomy to prevent diarrhea include dairy and legumes."
(D) "The colostomy should be irrigated at the same time everyday."

A–190

(A) Acromegaly is a disease that results from excess secretion of growth hormone usually caused by pituitary malignancies or malfunction. Clinical manifestations include increased sweating, decreased libido, mood disorders, muscle pain and weakness, moon-shaped face, enlarged feet and hands, deepened voice, and separation of the teeth. This condition often results in loss of vision. Small hands and feet and hearing loss are not known to be caused by acromegaly. Elephantiasis is massive swelling of lower parts of the body, particularly the genitalia and legs.

A–191

(A) After surgery to place a new colostomy, it normally takes an average of 3 to 6 days for the colostomy to begin functioning. To prevent skin irritation and irritation of the intestinal mucosa, a mild soap applied with a moist, soft cloth is used to clean the stoma. Diet is individualized to the nutritional needs of clients with colostomies. If a client experiences diarrhea, the food causing the diarrhea should be identified and eliminated. Irrigation aids in emptying the colon of gas, mucus, and feces. It is not necessary for every client with a colostomy to irrigate. If a client decides to irrigate, an individualized schedule for this procedure can be made by the client.

Q–192

During a seminar on cancer prevention, the community health nurse talks about risk factors associated with development of lung cancer. Select all of the following that would be included in this portion of the seminar as factors that predispose a person to lung cancer.

(A) Second-hand smoke inhalation
(B) Diet deficient in vitamin A
(C) Genetics
(D) Obesity
(E) Exposure to asbestos
(F) Race

Q–193

Mr. Franco returns to the hospital room following a bronchoscopy. His blood pressure is $\frac{135}{69}$, and his heart rate is in the 70s. Respirations are easy and unlabored. Still recovering from general anesthesia, Mr. Franco is resting in bed with his eyes closed. Which of the following physician's orders would the nurse question prior to initiating?

(A) Vital signs every 15 minutes for an hour, then routine
(B) Provide the client with ice chips
(C) Normal saline at 100 mL/hr
(D) Monitor the client on telemetry until further notice

Answers

A-192

(A), (B), (C), and (E) Predisposing factors that have been found to be associated with development of lung cancer include active and passive inhalation of tobacco smoke, environmental exposure to carcinogens (i.e., asbestos, radon), familial predisposition, and dietary factors such as low consumption of foods high in vitamin A. Obesity and race are not known to be related to development of cancer of the lung.

A-193

(B) The anesthesia used for a bronchoscopy procedure can range from a local anesthetic to general anesthesia. Most bronchoscopy procedures involve use of an agent to decrease discomfort in the throat and suppress the cough reflex. Until it is verified that the cough reflex is functioning, the client should not be offered anything by mouth, answer (B). Frequent vital signs for a given time period, fluid therapy, and telemetry monitoring are all appropriate physician's orders following this procedure.

Safe and Effective Care Environment:
Coordinated Care

Q–194

A client has a terminal form of cancer and is not expected to live more than a few weeks. Over the last few days, the client has been refusing pain medication because he says it makes him too sleepy and he wants to be alert to be with his family. The nurse believes the client needs the pain medication and administers the medication IV without informing the client. What value has the nurse used to perform this action?

(A) Paternalism
(B) Autonomy
(C) Beneficence
(D) Nonmaleficence

Safe and Effective Care Environment:
Coordinated Care

Q–195

Which situation would allow a client to have an invasive procedure without an informed consent being signed by the client or the client's parent or guardian?

(A) The client has broken both arms and is not able to write.
(B) The client has dementia and does not have any living family members.
(C) The client is an emancipated minor who refuses to sign any type of form.
(D) The client is unconscious and needs immediate surgery.

Answers

A–194

(A) Paternalism is to ignore the client's wishes (autonomy) and provide the client with what the nurse thinks is best in the situation. In this case, the nurse secretly gave the client pain medication even though the client did not want to take it. Beneficence is the duty to do or promote good, and nonmaleficence is the duty to do no harm.

A–195

(D) The only reason an informed consent is not signed is when the client is unconscious, there are no family members available, and the need for the procedure outweighs the need for consent to be signed. A client who is unable to write will be allowed to make an "X" instead of a signature. An emancipated minor must still sign consent forms before having a procedure. A client with dementia and no family will have a state guardian appointed who is responsible for signing informed consents.

Health Promotion and Maintenance

Q-196

A primagravid client at 38 weeks gestation comes to the labor and delivery department of the hospital saying that she has noticed an increase in vaginal discharge. The client denies noticing blood in the discharge. She is not experiencing any contractions. A nitrazine tape test is performed. The tape turns bluish-green. These results indicate

(A) the amniotic sac is probably broken.
(B) the amniotic sac is probably not broken.
(C) the cervix is ready for labor.
(D) the cervix is not ready for labor.

Health Promotion and Maintenance

Q-197

During a prenatal visit, the client states that she has been experiencing heartburn frequently. The LPN/LVN provides instruction on the cause and prevention of heartburn. When asked to verbalize understanding of the information, which of the following statements by the client indicates further instruction may be necessary?

(A) "The sphincter that normally prevents stomach contents from going back up into the esophagus is relaxed."
(B) "I should try to avoid drinking fluids while I'm eating."
(C) "Eating six or seven small meals a day may help my symptoms."
(D) "I'll eat enough to ensure that I am full at every meal."

Answers

(A) A nitrazine tape test is performed to identify the presence of amniotic fluid in vaginal discharge. The tape changes color according to the pH of the applied discharge. The color of the tape will change to bluish-green, bluish-gray, or a deep blue to indicate the pH of the discharge. False positives are possible. Therefore, these results indicate that the amniotic membranes have probably ruptured. Answer (A) is correct. Readiness of the cervix for labor is not indicated by this test.

(D) Heartburn in pregnancy is caused by an increase in the production of progesterone, which slows movement of stomach contents through the stomach and relaxes the cardiac sphincter. This allows reflux of food and gastric acid up into the esophagus to occur easily. Measures to prevent heartburn include avoiding fluids with meals, eating small and more frequent meals throughout the day, avoiding distention of the stomach by overeating, avoiding lying down for at least 30 minutes after a meal, and avoiding fatty or greasy foods. Answer (D) suggests that instruction might need to be reinforced on preventing stomach distention.

Health Promotion and Maintenance

Q–198

A 25-year-old client with diabetes mellitus Type I visits the clinic to discuss her and her husband's desire to start a family. This diabetic client

(A) should be discouraged from becoming pregnant.
(B) has a greater risk of complications during pregnancy.
(C) should be informed about treatment for infertility.
(D) will be able to carry out a completely normal pregnancy.

Health Promotion and Maintenance

Q–199

The nurse identifies substance abuse behaviors exhibited by a pregnant client during an initial prenatal screening. While promoting a therapeutic and accepting environment, the care management by the nurse would be most appropriate if focused on which of the following?

(A) Discouraging substance use during pregnancy
(B) Termination of the pregnancy at an early stage
(C) Eliminating substance use during pregnancy
(D) Setting boundaries with the client in regards to substance use

A-198

(B) Clients with diabetes mellitus are at greater risk for developing maternal and fetal complications during pregnancy. Answer (B) is correct. Risks to the neonate born to a diabetic mother are also more likely. However, many women who are pregestationally diabetic or become diabetic during gestation deliver healthy newborns with minimal or no complications. During pregnancy, labor, and following delivery, adjustments must be made to the diabetic client's normal regimen. Infertility is an issue separate from the existence of diabetes during pregnancy.

A-199

(C) Use of substances during pregnancy can lead to severe fetal or neonatal abnormalities, complications, and death. The primary goal of nursing care should be prevention of substance use during pregnancy. Discouraging substance use and/or setting boundaries with a client will not ensure prevention of the risks associated with even minimal substance use. Nursing actions that push the client to terminate the pregnancy are neither therapeutic nor appropriate to the client or the situation.

Health Promotion and Maintenance

Q–200

During a lecture on reproduction, a student nurse asks the instructor what determines the sex of a fetus. Accurate information in response to this question would be:

(A) "The sex of the fetus is not determined until the eighth week of gestation."
(B) "The fertilization of the zygote is the point at which sex is determined."
(C) "Males have one less pair of chromosomes than females."
(D) "Sex is determined by the chromosomes contributed by the ovum."

Health Promotion and Maintenance

Q–201

The LPN/LVN caring for newborns in the nursery notices a baby boy born 20 hours prior has an unusually high-pitched cry. The neonate is becoming increasingly irritable and restless. Later in the day, the newborn displays seizure activity. This neonate's condition suggests that his mother was addicted to which of the following during gestation?

(A) Heroin
(B) Cocaine
(C) Crack
(D) Marijuana

Answers

(B) The sex of the fetus is determined at the point that the sperm fertilizes the ovum to form the zygote, answer (B). This occurs within 72 hours after insemination. Males and females have an equal number of chromosomes. Both the sperm and the ovum contribute 23 chromosomes to form the zygote. The 23rd pair of chromosomes, one from the sperm and one from the ovum, determines the sex of the developing fetus. The ovum may only contribute an X chromosome. The sperm contributes either an X or a Y chromosome. Females have two X chromosomes. Males have an X and a Y chromosome. Therefore, sex is ultimately determined by the chromosome contributed by the sperm.

(A) Signs in a neonate that suggest maternal heroin addiction during pregnancy include restlessness, a shrill and high-pitched cry, irritability, fist sucking, vomiting, and seizures. Irritability, exaggerated startle reflex, and labile emotions of a neonate along with sudden infant death syndrome (SIDS) are associated with maternal use of cocaine while pregnant. Crack is a form of cocaine. Infants that were exposed to marijuana while in the uterus display fine tremors, prolonged startle reflexes, and irritability.

Physiological Integrity:
Basic Care and Comfort

Q–202

The nurse is taking the vital signs of an infant brought to the clinic for a routine well-child checkup. Which of the following describes the method for calculating the respiration rate of an infant?

(A) Count the number of respirations in a full minute.
(B) Count the number of respirations in 30 seconds and multiply by two.
(C) Count the number of respirations in 20 seconds and multiply by three.
(D) Count the number of respirations in 15 seconds and multiply by four.

Health Promotion and Maintenance

Q–203

The nurse assesses the development of a 13-month-old boy. Inability of the child to perform which of the following tasks indicates possible developmental delay?

(A) Stand alone
(B) Walk backwards
(C) Scribble on paper
(D) Play pat-a-cake

Answers

(A) Normal respirations by infants are often at an irregular rate. Therefore, to obtain the most accurate respiration rate, in respirations/min, the nurse should count the number of respirations in a full minute. For an older child or an adult, it is appropriate to count respirations in whatever fraction of a minute is desired. This number is then multiplied by the corresponding number to obtain respirations/min.

(D) According to the Denver II Developmental Screening Exam, 90% of children at the age of $11\frac{1}{2}$ months are able to play pat-a-cake. Inability to do so at 13 months indicates developmental delay. Between 75% and 85% of children are able to stand alone at the age of 13 months. About 35% of children are able to walk backwards at this child's age. Scribbling on paper is a task that about 40% of children are able to perform at the age of 13 months.

Physiological Integrity:
Pharmacological Therapies

Q–204

Pediazole is a suspension medication that contains 200 mg erythromycin and 600 mg sulfisoxazole per 5 mL. The physician orders Pediazole 4 mL p.o. every 12 hours. How many mg of sulfisoxazole is this client receiving in a 24-hour period?

(A) 160 mg
(B) 320 mg
(C) 480 mg
(D) 960 mg

Health Promotion and Maintenance

Q–205

The weight of a just-delivered newborn is 3050 grams (g). The nurse would convert this weight to pounds (lbs) to announce the baby's weight to the parents. The newborn's weight in pounds is _____.

Answers

(D) Solve for x mL per dose using the following calculations.

$$\frac{600 \text{ mg}}{5 \text{ mL}} = \frac{x \text{ mg}}{4 \text{ mL}}$$

$$2400 = 5x$$

$$x = \frac{2400}{5}$$

$$x = 480 \text{ mg per dose}$$

Determine amount given in 24 hours by multiplying the amount per dose in mg (480 mg) by the number of doses given in 24 hours (every 12 hours = 2). 480 × 2 = 960 mg in 24 hours. The correct answer is (D).

ANSWER: 6.7 lbs
RATIONALE: Use the following conversions to determine the weight in lbs.

$$1000 \text{ grams (g)} = 1 \text{ kg}$$

$$\frac{3050 \text{ g}}{1} = \frac{1 \text{ kg}}{1000 \text{ g}} = 3.05 \text{ kg}$$

$$1 \text{ kg} = 2.2 \text{ lbs}$$

$$\frac{3.05 \text{ kg}}{1} = \frac{2.2 \text{ lbs}}{1 \text{ kg}} = 6.7 \text{ lbs}$$

Health Promotion and Maintenance

Q–206

The LPN/LVN is caring for an 83-year-old client with Alzheimer's disease in an extended care facility. The client becomes confused at times, and the nurse also notices that the client's gait is unsteady. Select all of the following that would be appropriate nursing actions for the LPN/LVN to perform.

(A) Suggest to the physician and physical therapist that the client receive a walker for ambulating in the facility.
(B) Ask the family to bring in some of the client's belongings from home, such as knick-knacks and photos of friends and family members.
(C) Suggest that the client eat her meals in her room.
(D) Put up a clock and a calendar in the client's room.
(E) Encourage the client to ambulate by taking a walk in the hall twice a day.
(F) Apply soft wrist restraints to the client while in bed.

Health Promotion and Maintenance

Q–207

The LPN/LVN is caring for a 64-year-old client. The nurse would recognize that members of this age group deal with which of the following central tasks?

(A) Intimacy versus isolation
(B) Integrity versus despair
(C) Generativity versus stagnation
(D) Industry versus inferiority

Answers

(A), **(B)**, and **(D)** are correct answers. Nursing care for a client with Alzheimer's disease includes providing a calm, predictable daily routine and environment. Having familiar items such as photos of familiar people and displaying a calendar and a clock in the room will reduce sensory deprivation and decrease episodes of confusion. Eating alone or in a secluded environment will decrease stimulation, which may lead to sensory deprivation. Restraining the client may lead to an agitated state and should be avoided. This client has an unsteady gait. Use of a walker during ambulation will aid mobility. The client should not walk in the hall alone due to episodes of confusion.

(C) This client is in the stage of adulthood, ages 25 to 65. According to Erik Erikson's eight stages of development, the central developmental task of this stage is generativity versus stagnation. The resolution of the conflicts involved with each stage allows a person to function effectively in society. Intimacy versus isolation is the central task of the young adulthood stage, which includes ages 18 to 25. Integrity versus despair is the central task of the maturity stage, which includes ages 65 to death. Industry versus inferiority is the central task of the school-age stage, which includes ages 6 to 12.

Health Promotion and Maintenance

Q–208

According to Havighurst, select all of the following that are developmental tasks of the "middle adulthood" age period.

(A) Achieving adult civic responsibility
(B) Adjusting to aging parents
(C) Managing a home
(D) Learning to live with a partner
(E) Establishing an explicit affiliation with one's age group
(F) Developing appropriate leisure-time activities

Psychosocial Integrity

Q–209

The LPN/LVN overhears a student nurse conversing with a client. The client is expressing concern over her teenage son being home alone while she has been in the hospital. The student nurse replies, "Don't worry, everything will turn out all right." Which of the following communication tactics does this represent?

(A) Giving common advice
(B) Unwarranted reassurance
(C) Acknowledging
(D) Reflecting

Answers

(A), **(B)**, and **(F)** are the correct choices. According to Havighurst's developmental tasks, the "middle adulthood" age period involves: achieving adult civic and social responsibility; establishing and maintaining an economic standard of living; assisting teenage children to become responsible and happy adults; developing adult leisure-time activities; relating oneself to one's spouse as a person; accepting and adjusting to the physiologic changes of middle age; adjusting to aging parents. Managing a home and learning to live with a partner are tasks of "early adulthood." Establishing an explicit affiliation with one's age group is a task of "later maturity."

(B) Using clichés or comforting statements to reassure the client is a communication barrier called "unwarranted reassurance." These comments can block feelings and thoughts from a client. "Giving common advice," another communication barrier, is telling the client what to do in a situation. "Acknowledging" is recognizing a client behavior or effort in a nonjudgmental way. "Reflecting" involves directing ideas, feelings, or other content back to the client to allow exploration of a situation. "Acknowledging" and "reflecting" are therapeutic communication techniques.

Psychosocial Integrity

Q–210

A male client at the urgent care clinic has a broken hand. The client states that he became angry during an argument with his wife and punched the wall. Which of the following defense mechanisms would the LPN/LVN recognize this action as?

(A) Displacement
(B) Compensation
(C) Regression
(D) Sublimation

Psychosocial Integrity

Q–211

The nurse is caring for a client with bipolar disorder. Which meal would be most appropriate for this client during a manic episode?

(A) Spaghetti and meatballs with a salad
(B) Tomato soup, cheese slices, and an apple
(C) Tuna sandwich cut in quarters, carrot sticks, and orange slices
(D) Turkey with gravy, mashed potatoes, and peas

Answers

(A) Transferring emotional reaction from one person or thing to another person or thing is called displacement, answer (A). Compensation is accommodating for a weakness by overachievement or emphasizing a more desirable trait. Regression involves resorting to an earlier and more comfortable level of functioning. Sublimation is putting inappropriate or unacceptable energy into energy that is more acceptable.

(C) During the manic phase of bipolar disorder, a client has a high amount of energy. Nutritionally balanced finger food meals are preferred when choosing foods for this client because they don't require sitting still and focusing. The client can access the food throughout the day to meet high energy needs. The best answer choice is (C). All other choices involve foods that require sitting at the table to eat.

Psychosocial Integrity

Q–212

A client experiencing disorganized speech, poor contact with reality, and severe personality decompensation is admitted to the psychiatric unit. The client is hostile and shows signs of very little insight. Which of the following disorders should the LPN/LVN recognize these behaviors as exhibiting?

(A) Psychosis
(B) Neurosis
(C) Personality disorder
(D) Psychophysiological disorder

Physiological Integrity:
Basic Care and Comfort

Q–213

The nurse is preparing to provide care for a client's tracheostomy. Arrange the following choices in the correct order for carrying out this procedure.

(A) Clean the incision site and tube flange.
(B) Establish a sterile field.
(C) Using a sterile brush or pipe cleaners, clean the inner cannula.
(D) Suction the tracheostomy tube.
(E) Apply a sterile dressing.
(F) Remove the inner cannula.
(G) Replace the inner cannula.

A-212

(A) A client with psychosis exhibits alterations in one or more areas of normal functioning and displays a severe loss of contact with reality. Neurosis affects personality, mood, and some other areas of behavior but does not distract the client from performing normal activities. Personality disorder involves patterns of inflexible and maladaptive behavior, which can cause severe inability to function. Psychophysiological disorder involves physical symptoms caused or affected by emotional factors.

A-213

The appropriate order is **(B)**, **(D)**, **(F)**, **(A)**, **(C)**, **(G)**, and **(E)**. The correct procedure for tracheostomy care is as follows: prepare the client; establish a sterile field with all necessary equipment; don one clean glove on the nondominant hand to hold the tracheostomy, while suctioning the tracheostomy tube with the dominant sterile gloved hand; remove the inner cannula and place in soaking solution; remove the old dressing; apply sterile gloves to both hands; clean the incision site and tube flange; clean the presoaked inner cannula using a sterile brush; replace the inner cannula; and apply a sterile dressing.

Physiological Integrity:
Pharmacological Therapies

Q–214

The LPN/LVN has initiated the administration of vancomycin via IV piggyback. In which of the following situations should the nurse recognize that the client may be experiencing a fatal reaction to this medication?

(A) The client starts coughing.
(B) The client complains of pain at the intravenous catheter insertion site.
(C) The nurse hears the client snoring from the hall.
(D) The nurse notices the client's neck and chest is bright red.

Physiological Integrity:
Reduction of Risk Potential

Q–215

A 35-year-old client is visiting her physician for an annual gynecological exam. The client is in a monogamous relationship with her husband of 14 years. She is not complaining of any symptoms. The LPN/LVN notices a strong fishy odor during the vaginal exam. Which of the following would the nurse suspect the physician to test the client for?

(A) Urinary tract infection (UTI)
(B) Bacterial vaginosis (BV)
(C) Vulvovaginal candidiasis
(D) Trichomoniasis

Answers

A-214

(D) While administering vancomycin, the LPN/LVN should know to monitor the client carefully for the development of Red Man Syndrome. This condition is an anaphylactic reaction to vancomycin that displays as pruritis (itching), flushing, and erythema (redness) to the head, neck, and upper body. Coughing is not an adverse reaction to vancomycin, nor is it fatal. Pain at the IV catheter site is probably caused by localized tissue irritation and does not suggest a life-threatening situation. Snoring does not suggest a potentially fatal condition.

A-215

(B) Bacterial vaginosis is caused by overgrowth of bacteria normally found in the vagina. Over 50% of women with BV are asymptomatic. A characteristic fish-like odor is often used to identify BV when a client is asymptomatic. Urinary tract infections cause symptoms such as dysuria, frequency, and urgency. Symptoms of vulvovaginal cadidiasis, more commonly called a vaginal yeast infection, include a cheesy discharge, itching, and irritation to the vagina. Trichomoniasis is a sexually transmitted infection (STI) that often causes inflammation to the vagina.

Q–216

The physician prescribes Flagyl tid to a client with bacterial vaginosis (BV). The LPN/LVN reviews information about this medication with the client. Which of the following statements by the client would indicate that the client understood the instructions?

(A) "I understand the medication might leave a sour taste in my mouth."
(B) "I'll take the prescribed dose with each meal during the day."
(C) "If I miss a dose, I'll take two at once to make up for it."
(D) "I usually only drink one glass of wine a day with my dinner, but I'll avoid that until my prescription is finished."

Q–217

The physician has discussed methods for prevention of osteoporosis with an adult, female client. Which of the following types of exercise would be recommended to this client?

(A) Weight-bearing exercise
(B) Anaerobic exercise
(C) Isometric exercise
(D) Range-of-motion exercises

A–216

(D) Ingesting any amount of alcohol while on Flagyl can cause debilitating symptoms similar to exaggerated hangover symptoms. The client should be warned to avoid alcohol consumption for the duration of the prescription. Flagyl may leave a metallic taste in the mouth as opposed to a sour taste. The medication should be taken at equal intervals around the clock according to physician's orders, and the client should never take two doses of Flagyl at once.

A–217

(A) Bone growth and production is stimulated by weight-bearing activities, such as walking and skiing. Anaerobic exercise, such as weight lifting, is used for endurance training. Isometric exercise, used for immobilized joints, involves muscle tightening without moving the limb. Range-of-motion exercises are used to maintain or increase joint motion.

Q–218

The LPN/LVN student is presenting information to the class about osteoarthritis. Which of the following would NOT be included as a risk factor for osteoarthritis?

(A) Race
(B) Weight
(C) Age
(D) Gender

Physiological Integrity:
Basic Care and Comfort

Q–219

The LPN/LVN is assisting a quadriplegic client with passive range-of-motion exercises. The LPN/LVN moves the client's left leg away from the midline of the body. Which of the following range-of-motion exercises is this an example of?

(A) Adduction
(B) Abduction
(C) Pronation
(D) Eversion

A–218

(A) Risk factors for osteoarthritis, also known as degenerative joint disease, include increased age, genetic disposition, gender (females are more prone to osteoarthritis due to hormones and hormonal changes), obesity, mechanical factors (i.e., joint trauma, sports activities, and occupation), and prior inflammatory disease. The correct choice would be answer (A), which is not a factor that affects development of osteoarthritis.

A–219

(B) Movement away from the midline of the body is called abduction, answer (B). Adduction is the movement toward the midline of the body. Pronation is rotation of the forearm so that the palm of the hand is down. Eversion is a movement that turns the sole of the foot outward.

Health Promotion and Maintenance

Q–220

The physician places the palm of his hand at various positions on a client's back as the client repeatedly says "blue moon." This is representative of what assessment technique?

Physiological Integrity:
Pharmacological Therapies

Q–221

The LPN/LVN is preparing to administer Solu-medrol 40 mg mixed in 150 ml of sodium chloride via intravenous piggyback. The medication is to be administered over 30 minutes. Using tubing with a drop factor of 15 gtt/mL, what would the LPN/LVN calculate the rate to be in drops per minute?

(A) 40
(B) 50
(C) 75
(D) 150

Answers

ANSWER: Tactile fremitus
RATIONALE: Tactile fremitus is an assessment technique used to test density and uniformity of the lungs. Fremitus, a palpable vibration, occurs from sound traveling from the larynx to the wall of the chest or back. Increased or decreased fremitus indicates abnormalities. A discrepancy in fremitus of various lung fields also indicates possible pulmonary disease.

(C) The formula to calculate this problem is: x gtt/min = volume/time (in minutes) × drop factor.

$$x \text{ gtt/min} = \frac{150 \text{ mL}}{30 \text{ min}} \times 15 \text{ gtt/min}$$

$$x \text{ gtt/min} = 75$$

The correct answer is (C).

Physiological Integrity:
Physiological Adaptation

Q–222

Mr. Nelson, an 82-year-old client, is admitted to the hospital after sustaining a fall on his front porch steps. While assisting the client with morning care, the nurse notes brownish discoloration on the medial malleolus of both ankles. Which of the following should the LPN/LVN recognize this to be a sign of?

(A) Elder abuse
(B) Tinea corporis
(C) Normal skin changes with age
(D) Venous insufficiency

Health Promotion and Maintenance

Q–223

Which of the following are recommendations for cancer screening of asymptomatic people, according to the American Cancer Society? Select all that apply.

(A) Digital rectal exam annually beginning at age 40 (males and females).
(B) Monthly breast self-examination beginning at age 20 (females).
(C) Digital rectal prostate exam annually beginning at age 50 (males).
(D) Mammogram annually beginning at age 40 (females).
(E) Prostate-specific antigen blood test annually beginning at age 50 (males).
(F) Skin exam every 3 years over age 20.
(G) Thyroid exam annually over age 40.

A–222

(D) Venous insufficiency is a result of the ineffective function of venous valves in the legs, which causes venous stasis. Ulcers form from rupture of small skin veins and cause brown pigmentation of the skin most commonly found at the medial malleolus of the ankle. Other symptoms of venous insufficiency include pain, edema, and dermatitis at the site. This finding suggests a medical condition as opposed to elder abuse. Tinea corporis or ringworm infection of the body appears as a red macule that spreads into a ring of papules. This pigmentation should be recognized as a sign of a medical condition and not merely normal skin changes caused by age.

A–223

(A) through (G) are all correct answers. All of the above are the recommendations provided by the American Cancer Society to prevent the development of malignancies. These tests promote early detection since they are performed prior to symptoms occurring. Besides these areas, the American Cancer Society has recommended guidelines for asymptomatic people to prevent development of cervical and uterine cancer, testicular cancer, ovarian cancer, cancer of the lymph nodes, and cancer of the mouth and throat.

Physiological Integrity:
Basic Care and Comfort

Q–224

A client is receiving continuous nasogastric tube feeding. Which of the following is the best position for this client?

(A) Fowler's position
(B) Sim's position
(C) Lateral position
(D) Slightly elevated, right side-lying

Physiological Integrity:
Basic Care and Comfort

Q–225

A client is receiving continuous feedings through a gastric tube. The LPN/LVN has the formula set at a rate of 130 mL per hour with gastric residuals being checked every 4 hours as ordered by the physician. The nurse obtains a residual of 90 mL. Which of the following would be appropriate for the LPN/LVN to do at this time?

(A) Return the residual to the stomach and continue the tube feeding as before.
(B) Discard the residual and continue the tube feeding as before.
(C) Return the residual to the stomach and stop the tube feeding.
(D) Discard the residual and stop the tube feeding.

Answers

(A) To enhance gravitational flow through the gastrointestinal tract and prevent aspiration of fluid into the lungs, the proper position for a client receiving continuous tube feedings would be Fowler's position, answer (A). In Fowler's position the bed is kept between a 15° and a 90° angle. The angle can be adjusted for client comfort and to obtain the most normal sitting position for the client. If this position is not possible, the next most appropriate position would be a slightly elevated, right side-lying position, which promotes gastric emptying. Sim's and lateral positions both consist of the client in a side-lying position with the bed flat. Neither of these is appropriate during tube feedings.

(C) Residual feeding pulled from the stomach contains hydrochloric acid and gastric enzymes. To promote normal function, these stomach contents should not be removed from the stomach unless absolutely necessary. If the gastric residual is less than 150 mL, it should be returned to the stomach. If the gastric residual is more than 50% of the total feeding administered in the past hour, the feeding should be stopped until appropriate gastric motility is ensured. In this scenario, the gastric residual is less than 150 mL, and the residual is more than half of the amount administered in an hour. The correct answer is (C).

Questions

Physiological Integrity:
Basic Care and Comfort

Q–226

After using crutches for two weeks following surgical repair of a right femur fracture, Mr. Daniels has progressed to using a cane. While teaching the client how to properly use a standard cane for maximum support of the weak side, which of the following is correct instruction?

(A) Hold the cane with the right hand.
(B) While standing still, the tip of the cane should be 3 inches to the side and 3 inches in front of the foot.
(C) Move the cane forward about 1 foot.
(D) Move the cane and the weak leg forward at the same time.

Physiological Integrity:
Basic Care and Comfort

Q–227

T. McNair is an eight-year-old pediatric client in a spica cast. The LPN/LVN notices the client eats large amounts of food very rapidly at a meal. Following the meal the client complains of feeling uncomfortable. Which of the following would be an appropriate intervention for preventing this problem?

(A) Provide small, frequent meals to the client.
(B) Remove items from the client's meal tray prior to bringing it in the room.
(C) Put the client on a fluid restriction.
(D) Distract the client during meals to prevent rapid consumption.

A–226

(C) The cane should be held with the hand on the side of the body that the strong leg is on. In this case, the strong side is the left side. While standing, the tip of the cane should be positioned 6 inches to the side and 6 inches in front of the foot of the strong leg. When using the cane requires maximum support, the cane should be moved forward about 1 foot, and then the weak leg should be moved towards the cane while maintaining weight on the good leg. Once less support is needed due to strengthening of the affected leg, the cane and the weak leg can move together during use.

A–227

(A) The client should be offered small, frequent meals to ensure that his nutritional needs are met, while preventing bloating from eating too much too quickly. Withholding food from a client, especially a pediatric client who has high caloric needs is inappropriate. A fluid restriction could lead to constipation, which is already a risk factor for clients in spica casts. Distraction is not the most effective means of preventing this problem.

Q–228

The nurse is caring for a client who was admitted with diabetic ketoacidosis. As the client is recovering, he tells the nurse, "Please don't tell anyone, but I keep a stash of chocolate cupcakes in a closet. When no one is around, I eat one or two. I guess I went a little crazy this time." What is the best response by the nurse?

(A) "Don't worry. This will be our little secret."
(B) "Because this involves your health, I need to share this fact with your healthcare provider."
(C) "I'm going to write it in your chart, but that is the furthest it will go."
(D) "This involves your health. I need to tell your family to go clean out that closet."

Q–229

A nurse witnesses a serious motor vehicle accident and stops to offer assistance. An adult male is screaming for someone to help him. The nurse notes that the airbag has deployed and there is blood on the individual and inside the car. What is the nurse's best action for this accident victim?

(A) Attempt to extricate the victim from the car.
(B) Call for emergency assistance and stay with the victim.
(C) Look for the bleeding site and attempt to stop the bleeding.
(D) Find a sharp object and deflate the air bag.

Answers

A–228

(B) The client has to believe that there is privacy in what is revealed in conversations with the nurse. But the nurse has the duty to inform the healthcare provider about information that may compromise the client's health. In this case, the client is eating a lot of chocolate cupcakes and this may impact the way the healthcare provider plans for the client's home care. The nurse would not write it in the chart because this may be seen by other healthcare workers who do not need the information. It is also not the nurse's responsibility to inform the family.

A–229

(B) A nurse who witnesses an accident can only provide assistance that is within the scope of the nurse's practice and must not cause further injury to the accident victim. The best course of action is for the nurse to call 911 and stay with the victim until emergency assistance arrives. The nurse should not remove the victim from the vehicle unless the vehicle is on fire and shouldn't move the victim within the vehicle or make any changes to the vehicle unless it is affecting the victim's survival.

Physiological Integrity:
Pharmacological Therapies

Q–230

The physician orders ferrous sulfate (Feosol) 1 tablet p.o. tid for a client with iron deficiency anemia. Based on what the LPN/LVN knows about the absorption of this medication, the best time for administration would be which of the following times?

(A) One hour after meals
(B) With meals
(C) At regularly scheduled intervals
(D) One hour before meals

Safe and Effective Care Environment:
Coordinated Care

Q–231

A nurse has been "floated" to another unit. Upon arriving at that unit, the nurse is given an assignment. The nurse says to charge nurse, "There is no way I can handle all of these clients." I'm going back to my own unit. What charges may this nurse face? Select all that apply.

(A) Malpractice
(B) Abandonment
(C) Assault
(D) Slander
(E) Libel

Answers

A-230

(D) Ferrous sulfate (Feosol) is used to supplement iron in the body. Oral preparations of iron supplements are most effectively absorbed if administered 1 hour before or 2 hours after meals. This is because this mineral absorbs best on an empty stomach. Answer (D) is the best answer choice. The stomach would not be adequately emptied if the medication was given only one hour after the meals. If the client is unable to take this medication on an empty stomach, it can be given with meals to prevent gastric irritation. Regularly scheduled intervals do not ensure that the medication is given on an empty stomach.

A-231

(A) and (B) A nurse may not leave clients until it has been arranged for someone else to care for them. The nurse has not given care to a client so the nurse cannot be charged with assault. The nurse has not spoken or written about any of the clients, so there cannot be any charge of slander or libel. Malpractice is the failure of a healthcare professional to use ordinary or reasonable care or the failure to act in a reasonable and prudent manner. Leaving the floor without coverage is neither reasonable nor prudent.

Q–232

State law requires that all clients at an extended stay facility be tested for tuberculosis exposure. The purified protein derivative (PPD) is administered to the clients by the LPNs/LVNs. Which of the following represents an appropriate time for the results of this test to be checked following administration?

(A) 24 hours
(B) 48 hours
(C) One week
(D) Two weeks

Q–233

A client undergoes a total laryngectomy after diagnosis of laryngeal cancer. Which of the following would indicate compromise to the client's respiratory status following this surgery?

(A) Shivering
(B) Half-dollar-sized amount of blood drainage on bandage over incision
(C) Restlessness
(D) Oxygen saturation of 95%

Answers

A–232

(B) The purified protein derivative (PPD) is injected into the intradermal layer of the inner aspect of the forearm. The test results are read 48 to 72 hours after injection. The correct answer is (B). Twenty-four hours is too soon to check the results of this test. The results at this time would not give accurate indication of exposure. Whether or not tuberculosis exposure had occurred could not be determined from examining the site one or two weeks following the injection. These choices are too long after injection.

A–233

(C) Hypoxia caused by respiratory compromise would display the following signs: restlessness; rapid and shallow breathing; flaring nares; use of accessory muscles for breathing; hypertension; confusion; and cyanosis of the nail beds, lips, and skin. If not corrected, hypoxia will lead to coma and eventually death. The correct answer is (C), restlessness. Bloody drainage is expected following surgery. Shivering is a normal response following general anesthesia and surgery. The client should be offered another blanket. Oxygen saturation is the percentage of hemoglobin in the blood that is saturated with oxygen. Normal oxygen saturation is 95% to 100%.

Physiological Integrity:
Pharmacological Therapies

Q–234

The physician orders epinephrine 0.1 mg subcutaneously ×
1 now. The constitution of epinephrine according to the vial
is 1:1000, or 1 g of epinephrine per 1,000 mL of solution.
How much solution should be drawn into a syringe by the
LPN/LVN?

(A) 0.01 mL
(B) 0.1 mL
(C) 1.0 mL
(D) 10 mL

Physiological Integrity:
Pharmacological Therapies

Q–235

A female client visits the physician's office with complaints
of dysuria, frequency, and urgency. After diagnostic testing,
the client is told that she has a urinary tract infection (UTI).
Which of the following anti-infective classifications would
most likely be prescribed for this client?

(A) Sulfonamides
(B) Tetracyclines
(C) Aminoglycosides
(D) Vancomycin

Answers

(B) 1 gram epinephrine is equal to 1000 mg epinephrine. Solve for x mL using the following ratio method.

$$\frac{1000 \text{ mg}}{1000 \text{ mL}} = \frac{0.1 \text{ mg}}{x \text{ mL}}$$

$$1000x = 100$$

$$x = \frac{100}{1000}$$

$$x = 0.1 \text{ mL}$$

The correct answer is (B), 0.1 mL.

(A) Sulfonamides such as trimethoprim-sulfamethoxazole (Bactrim) are used to treat UTIs because of their effectiveness at reducing fecal, vaginal, and periurethral bacteria. Tetracyclines are most commonly used to treat acne and many sexually transmitted infections (STIs) such as gonorrhea, syphilis, and chlamydia. Aminoglycosides are most commonly used to treat infections of the gastrointestinal tract and tuberculosis. Vancomycin, which is an anti-infective in its own classification group, is commonly used to treat pneumonia, septicemia, endocarditis, and osteomyelitis.

Physiological Integrity:
Reduction of Risk Potential

Q–236

The LPN/LVN is reviewing a client's morning laboratory findings. The nurse notes that the client's serum creatinine level is elevated. Which of the following systems does this diagnostic test show the function of?

(A) Cardiovascular
(B) Renal
(C) Hepatic
(D) Pulmonary

Health Promotion and Maintenance

Q–237

The LPN/LVN is instructing a 21-year-old female client on how to perform a self-breast examination. Which of the following is NOT a correct statement regarding this exam?

(A) "You should perform this exam once a month."
(B) "Use the fingertips to palpate the breast tissue for abnormalities."
(C) "To thoroughly assess the breast tissue, it is recommended to perform the exam while in the shower, while standing in front of a mirror, and while lying down."
(D) "It is best to perform the exam one week before the menses begins."

Answers

(B) Serum creatinine is used diagnostically to show the function of the kidneys, or the renal function, answer (B). Creatinine is a byproduct of protein or muscle. Normal creatinine serum levels range from 0.6 to 1.2 mg/dL. Multiple tests are used to monitor the various functions of the lungs and heart (or pulmonary and cardiovascular systems). The test used depends on what specific function of these systems is being looked at. Serum creatinine does not show pulmonary or cardiovascular function. Hepatic function is usually tested by looking at serum levels of the enzymes that are excreted by the liver.

(D) It is recommended for women to begin performing monthly self-breast examinations around the age of 20 years old. It is recommended to perform the exam while in the shower, while standing in front of a mirror, and while lying down in order to thoroughly check the breast tissue for abnormalities. The fingertips are used to palpate the breast tissue because they are very sensitive and can most easily detect abnormalities. The best time of month to perform the exam is one week following the beginning of menstruation, making answer (D) correct.

Physiological Integrity:
Basic Care and Comfort

Q–238

Mrs. Tomlinson is diagnosed with benign fibrocystic disease of the breasts. The LPN/LVN informs the client that eliminating which of the following from her diet may help reduce the symptoms of this disorder?

(A) Cola
(B) Chocolate
(C) Carbohydrates
(D) Caffeine

Health Promotion and Maintenance

Q–239

Following a vasectomy, the LPN/LVN is providing discharge instructions to the client and his wife. Which of the following would be appropriate for the nurse to tell the couple?

(A) "The vasectomy makes you sterile."
(B) "After ten days you never have to use a condom again."
(C) "You will need to use an alternate birth control method for six weeks."
(D) "After six months you will be sterile."

A-238

(**D**) Caffeine is reported to contribute to the discomfort associated with benign fibrocystic disease of the breasts, answer (D). Although cola and chocolate do contain caffeine, caffeine must usually be avoided from all sources in order to decrease the symptoms. Carbohydrates are not known to contribute to the manifestations of this condition.

A-239

(**C**) Six weeks following the vasectomy, the sperm count will be checked. If the sperm count is zero, conception is nearly impossible. The sperm count is rechecked at six months and then every year. A vasectomy does not guarantee sterility. Ending use of a second birth control method ten days following the procedure is too soon to prevent conception.

Safe and Effective Care Environment:
Safety and Infection Control

Q–240

A client with syphilis shows symptoms of advancement of the disease to the tertiary stage. Which of the following clinical manifestations support this advancement? (Select all that apply.)

(A) Inflammation of the aorta
(B) Dementia
(C) Paresis
(D) Meningitis
(E) Stroke

Safe and Effective Care Environment:
Safety and Infection Control

Q–241

During a presentation by a student LPN/LVN on the major forms of viral hepatitis, which of the following would NOT be included as a risk for infection by hepatitis C?

(A) Frequent blood transfusion
(B) Contaminated drinking water
(C) IV drug needle sharing
(D) Sexual activity with multiple partners

Answers

(A) through (E) are all correct. Aortitis (inflammation of the aorta) and neurosyphilis are the most common manifestations of tertiary syphilis. Dementia, psychosis, paresis (partial paralysis), stroke, and meningitis are all associated with neurosyphilis. All of the answers above are correct. Syphilis advances to this tertiary stage in 60% to 80% of those infected with the disease.

(B) The hepatitis C virus is transmitted most commonly through blood transmissions and sexual activity with multiple partners. Sharing intravenous drug needles is also a very common mode of transmission for this virus. Health-care workers are at risk for infection with this virus due to accidental needle sticks. Drinking contaminated water is a mode of transmission for hepatitis A. Answer (B) is the correct choice.

Health Promotion and Maintenance

Q–242

A couple is visiting the obstetrician for a family-planning visit. They have decided to begin trying to conceive their first child. Which of the following would be appropriate for the LPN/LVN to instruct the husband to avoid?

(A) Wearing boxer shorts
(B) Sitting in a hot tub
(C) Eating spicy foods
(D) Swimming in a public pool

Physiological Integrity:
Pharmacological Therapies

Q–243

A pregnant client is admitted to the hospital with preeclampsia. The physician orders that the client be placed on magnesium sulfate via IV piggyback. The client begins to exhibit signs of magnesium toxicity. Which of the following would be administered immediately?

(A) Calcium gluconate (Kalcinate)
(B) Calcitonin (Calcimar)
(C) Terbutaline (Bricanyl)
(D) Oxytocin (Pitocin)

A–242

(**B**) Heat can damage or kill sperm. Therefore, while trying to conceive, it is advised that males avoid the use of hot tubs or taking baths. It would probably also be suggested that the husband wear loose-fitting clothes, including boxer shorts as opposed to underwear briefs. This allows air flow to the testes to decrease the temperature. Eating spicy foods and swimming in public pools will not affect sperm viability.

A–243

(**A**) Calcium is the antidote for serum magnesium excess. Calcium gluconate (Kalcinate) is a form of calcium that is given to reverse effects of excessive IV magnesium administration. Calcitonin (Calcimar) is the hormone that decreases levels of calcium in the blood by transferring it to the bone. Terbutaline (Bricanyl) is used to manage preterm labor. Oxytocin (Pitocin) is a hormone that stimulates uterine contraction and is used to induce labor.

Q–244

Serious conditions can develop as side effects of intravenous (IV) magnesium sulfate administration. The LPN/LVN is aware that which of the following should be carefully assessed during IV administration of magnesium sulfate to monitor for these serious conditions? (Select all that apply.)

(A) Respirations
(B) Urinary output
(C) Temperature
(D) Patellar tendon reflex
(E) Sense of smell
(F) Hearing

Health Promotion and Maintenance

Q–245

During her first prenatal visit, a 23-year-old pregnant client asks the LPN/LVN what would be normal weight gain for pregnancy. Considering the client was not overweight or underweight prior to becoming pregnant, normal weight gain would be between _____ and _____lbs.

Answers

A–244

(A), (B), and (D) are correct. Signs that toxicity is developing from intravenous (IV) magnesium sulfate administration include depression of reflexes, oliguria, confusion, respiratory depression or paralysis, and circulatory collapse. Deep tendon reflexes (i.e., patellar tendon reflex), blood pressure, heart rate, respirations, urinary output, and fetal heart tones should be closely monitored. Common side effects that are considered normal from magnesium sulfate administration include lethargy and weakness, sweating, flushing, nasal congestion, nausea, constipation, visual blurring, headaches, and slurred speech. These effects should subside once the medication is discontinued. Changes in temperature, sense of smell, and hearing are not known to develop from magnesium sulfate administration.

A–245

ANSWER: 25 to 35 lbs or 11 to 16 kg
RATIONALE: Weight gain is individualized during pregnancy depending on the person. If the client is underweight prior to pregnancy, it is recommended that she gain 28 to 40 lbs or 12.5 to 18 kg. If the client is overweight prior to pregnancy, she should gain between 15 and 25 lbs or 7 to 11.5 kg. Obese clients are recommended to gain no more than 15 lbs or 7 kg during pregnancy. A woman who is normal weight-for-height prior to pregnancy should gain between 25 and 35 lbs or 11 to 16 kg.

Health Promotion and Maintenance

Q–246

Which of the following is the recommended caloric intake for most women who are nursing?

(A) 1800 to 2000 kcal/day
(B) 2000 to 2200 kcal/day
(C) 2500 to 2700 kcal/day
(D) 3000 kcal/day

Health Promotion and Maintenance

Q–247

A laboratory technician enters the pediatric floor playroom to obtain a blood sample from a seven-year-old client. Which of the following would be an appropriate intervention for the LPN/LVN?

(A) Allow the technician to obtain the sample while the child is distracted with play.
(B) Explain to the child what will happen and ask if it is okay.
(C) Assist the technician to help hurry the process.
(D) Tell the technician that procedures are not allowed in the playroom.

Answers

A-246

(C) A woman's necessary caloric intake increases while nursing, even more so than during pregnancy. It is recommended that women increase caloric intake by 200 kcal above the requirements during pregnancy. This increase is about 500 kcal above pre-pregnancy requirements. For most nursing women this totals between 2500 and 2700 kcal/day, answer (C). Insufficient caloric intake can reduce milk volume. 1800 to 2200 kcal/day is the approximate range for caloric intake of a non-pregnant person. 3000 kcal/day is excessive of the caloric requirements while nursing.

A-247

(D) Hospitalized children need to have a place that is considered safe in the hospital environment. The playroom is considered safe, and procedures are not allowed in this room. Many hospitals have a "treatment room" where procedures are performed, leaving the child's room and bed as additional "safe places." This invasive procedure should never be performed in a "safe place" such as the playroom. Answer (D) is correct.

Physiological Integrity:
Basic Care and Comfort

Q–248

A four-year-old child is experiencing pain following a bone marrow aspiration procedure. Medication has been administered and the LPN/LVN is attempting to use play as a diversion technique. Which of the following toys would be *least* appropriate for the nurse to use for a child at this developmental level?

(A) Books containing different textures
(B) Building blocks
(C) Play carpentry tools
(D) Crayons

Physiological Integrity:
Pharmacological Therapies

Q–249

Amanda is a seven-year-old client on methylphenidate (Ritalin) for attention deficit hyperactivity disorder (ADHD). Which of the following statements from her mother would indicate that changes should be made to Amanda's medication regimen?

(A) "Amanda got 90% on her last spelling test."
(B) "Amanda hasn't eaten much of the lunches I've packed for her lately."
(C) "Amanda goes to sleep at 9 P.M. in order to get up in time for school the next day."
(D) "Amanda had a sleepover last Saturday night."

Answers

(A) Preschool-aged children require toys that provide stimulation of fine motor skills and self-expression. At this age, manipulative and constructive toys are best to promote quiet activities. These toys include multi-shaped building blocks, paints, crayons, play carpentry/sewing/cooking/construction toys, large puzzles, and clay. Books with different textures are more appropriate for infants and toddlers. Answer (A) is the correct choice.

(B) Answer (B) indicates that Amanda is experiencing a decrease in appetite as a side effect of this medication and is therefore the correct answer. Other side effects include insomnia and nervousness. Positive effects from the use of methylphenidate (Ritalin) include self-confidence, increased socialization, and improvement in schoolwork. Answers (A) and (D) represent positive effects of Ritalin. Sleeping from around 9 P.M. until it is time to get up for school suggests the absence of insomnia.

Physiological Integrity:
Basic Care and Comfort

Q–250

A hospitalized child weighs 28 lbs. The physician orders maintenance fluids for this child. What would the LPN/LVN calculate to be the daily IV fluid volume for this child?

(A) 1660 mL daily
(B) 1135 mL daily
(C) 775 mL daily
(D) 554 mL daily

Physiological Integrity:
Physiological Adaptation

Q–251

Which of the following assessment findings of a ten-day-old neonate would support a diagnosis of coarctation of the aorta?

(A) Bounding femoral pulses
(B) Weakness in the legs
(C) Higher blood pressure in the right arm than the right leg
(D) Circumoral cyanosis

A-250

(B) Pediatric daily IV fluid maintenance volume would be calculated using the following formula: (100 mL/kg/day for the first 10 kg) + (50 mL/kg/day for the next 10 kg) + (20 mL/kg/day for each kg above 20 kg).

$$\frac{28 \text{ lb}}{2.2 \text{ kg}} = 12.7 \text{ kg}$$

10 kg (100 mL) + 2.7 kg (50 mL) = 1135 mL daily
Answer (B) is correct.

A-251

(C) Coarctation of the aorta is a congenital heart defect where there is a narrowing at some point in the aorta. Clinical manifestations include high blood pressure and bounding pulses in the upper extremities with low blood pressure and weak or absent pulses in the lower extremities, answer (C). This condition can lead to rapid hemodynamic deterioration. Weakness in the legs and circumoral cyanosis (bluish coloring around the mouth) may eventually appear from this condition. However, these are symptoms more commonly associated with other conditions.

Health Promotion and Maintenance

Q–252

Arrange the following cognitive stages of development as defined by Piaget from youngest to oldest.

(A) Formal operations
(B) Concrete operations
(C) Preoperational thought, intuitive phase
(D) Preoperational thought, preconceptual phase
(E) Sensorimotor

Health Promotion and Maintenance

Q–253

A 30-month-old boy is brought to the clinic by his mother who suspects that he has an ear infection. Which of the following is a correct technique when assessing the internal ear of this child with an otoscope?

(A) Pull the earlobe down
(B) Pull the pinna (upper curve) of the ear up
(C) Pull the pinna (upper curve) of the ear back
(D) Pull the pinna (upper curve) of the ear down

A-252

(E), **(D)**, **(C)**, **(B)**, and **(A)**. According to Jean Piaget, a child will mature through development following these stages: sensorimotor (from birth to 2 years); preoperational thought, preconceptual phase using transductive reasoning (from 2 to 4 years); preoperational thought, intuitive phase using transductive reasoning (from 4 to 7 years); concrete operations using inductive reasoning and beginning logic (7 to 11 years); formal operations using deductive and abstract reasoning (from 11 to 15 years).

A-253

(D) The canal of the inner ear is in the shape of the letter "S." In order to straighten this curve, the pinna (upper curve) of the ear of an infant or child younger than three years old would be pulled down. For children older than three years old and adults, the ear is pulled back. There are no circumstances in which the pinna would be pulled up or the ear lobe would be pulled down.

Health Promotion and Maintenance

Q–254

The LPN/LVN is providing discharge instructions to the parents of a six-year-old who just had a tonsillectomy. Which of the following would the nurse alert the parents to watch for as a sign of excessive bleeding?

(A) Frequent swallowing
(B) Low-grade fever
(C) Mild ear pain
(D) Foul odor from the mouth

Physiological Integrity:
Reduction of Risk Potential

Q–255

A five-year-old child is admitted to the hospital with pneumococcal pneumonia. The child is placed on continuous pulse oximetry. To indicate appropriate respiratory status, this reading should stay at or above what value?

Answers

A–254

(A) An early sign that is the most indicative of excessive bleeding following a tonsillectomy is continuous swallowing, answer (A). This indicates that blood is trickling in the back of the throat. It is normal to experience a low-grade fever, mild ear pain, and mouth odor for a few days following a tonsillectomy. Persistence of these symptoms would require medical follow-up.

A–255

ANSWER: 95%
RATIONALE: Pulse oximetry measures the amount of oxygen saturated in the blood. A reading of 95% or higher indicates sufficient oxygen supply to the organs of the body. Intervention is necessary if the value goes below 95%.

Q–256

Keflex 500 mg p.o. every 6 hours is prescribed for a child admitted to the pediatric floor for treatment of pneumonia. The nurse asks the mother if the child has ever had an allergic reaction to a medication. An allergic reaction to which of the following medications would indicate that the nurse should clarify this order with the physician?

(A) Tetracycline
(B) Amoxicillin
(C) Gentamicin
(D) Vancomycin

Q–257

Mr. Sheffield is placed on a fluid restriction and daily weights for congestive heart failure (CHF). Mr. Sheffield's intake for the past 24 hours is approximately 2500 mL. The client's output for the past 24 hours is approximately 1500 mL. Which of the following trends would the nurse expect to see in the client's weight?

(A) Mr. Sheffield's weight increased by 1 lb from yesterday to today.
(B) Mr. Sheffield's weight was 152.2 lb yesterday and is 154.4 lb today.
(C) Mr. Sheffield's weight was 69.2 kg yesterday and is 71.4 kg today.
(D) There is no change in Mr. Sheffield's weight from yesterday to today.

Answers

(B) Keflex is a first-generation cephalosporin, which is used to treat infections. Cephalosporins are known to cause allergic reactions in clients who have had allergic reactions to penicillins in the past. Amoxicillin is a penicillin anti-infective. Tetracycline is a tetracycline anti-infective. Gentamicin is an aminoglycoside anti-infective. Vancomycin is in its own category of anti-infective. Tetracyclines, aminoglycosides, and vancomycin are not known to cause cross-reactions with cephalosporins.

(B) The 24-hour I & O's reflect that Mr. Sheffield has retained approximately 1000 mL or 1 L of fluid. Mr. Sheffield's weight should have increased equivalent to the weight of one liter of fluid, which is 1 kg or 2.2 lb. Answer (A) shows only a 1-lb increase in weight. Answer (C) shows a 2.2-kg increase in weight as opposed to pounds. Answer (D) is incorrect because the client's weight should have changed over the 24-hour period.

Q–258

A client is receiving a continuous heparin drip infusion at 1000 units/hr. Following the most recent PTT results, the physician orders that the infusion rate be increased to 1200 units/hr. The composition of medication in solution is 50,000 units of heparin in 500 mL D_5W. Which of the following represents the change in mL/hr from the old to the new rate?

(A) 1000 mL/hr increased to 1200 mL/hr

(B) 500 mL/hr increased to 700 mL/hr

(C) 10 mL/hr increased to 12 mL/hr

(D) 100 mL/hr increased to 120 mL/hr

Answers

(C) Solve for x mL/hr using the following ratio method.

$$\frac{50,000 \text{ units}}{500 \text{ mL}} = \frac{1000 \text{ units}}{x \text{ mL}}$$

$$50,000x = 500,000$$

$$x = \frac{500,000}{50,000}$$

$$x = 10 \text{ mL/hr (old rate)}$$

$$\frac{50,000 \text{ units}}{500 \text{ mL}} = \frac{1200 \text{ units}}{x \text{ mL}}$$

$$50,000x = 600,000$$

$$x = \frac{600,000}{50,000}$$

$$x = 12 \text{ mL/hr (new rate)}$$

The correct answer is (C).

Physiological Integrity:
Pharmacological Therapies

Q–259

The LPN/LVN is volunteering at a local facility that is providing tuberculosis (TB) screening to indigent community members. Select all of the following factors that increase risk for TB infection.

(A) Recent travel to an Asian country
(B) Recent hospitalization for pneumonia
(C) Sexual activity with multiple partners
(D) Chemotherapy treatment for cancer
(E) Close contact with someone who tested positive for TB exposure
(F) Psychiatric facility members

Physiological Integrity:
Pharmacological Therapies

Q–260

There are many medications used to treat pulmonary tuberculosis (TB) infection. Which of the following medications is NOT used for this purpose?

(A) 3TC
(B) Rifampin
(C) Ethambutol
(D) Streptomycin

A-259

(A), (D), and (F) are correct. Tuberculosis (TB) is spread by airborne transmission. Risk factors for tuberculosis (TB) infection include close contact with someone who has active TB, immunocompromised status (i.e., clients with HIV, cancer, organ transplants, or long-term steroidal therapy), substance abuse, pre-existing medical conditions or special treatments, travel to or immigration from countries with high TB prevalence (i.e., Asia, Africa, Latin America, Caribbean), institutionalization, healthcare workers in high-risk airborne transmission activities, and living in substandard housing. Pneumonia does not lead to TB. TB is not transmitted sexually. TB is only transmitted from those with active TB. Testing positive for TB exposure does not mean the TB is active.

A-260

(A) Medications used to treat tuberculosis (TB) include isoniazid (INH), rifampin, streptomycin, pyrazinamide, and ethambutol. It is also common for combination therapy, usually with rifampin and INH, to be used. Lamivudine or 3TC is an antiretroviral medication used to slow progression of HIV and decrease the occurrence of secondary infections due to immunocompromised status.

The LPN/LVN is preparing to assist a client with right-sided hemiplegia following a cerebrovascular accident (CVA) to transfer from the bed to a wheelchair. Which of the following is appropriate for the nurse to do during this activity?

(A) Place the wheelchair perpendicular to the bed.
(B) Place the wheelchair parallel to the bed on the client's left side.
(C) Place the wheelchair parallel to the bed on the client's right side.
(D) Stand behind the wheelchair to stabilize.

Q–262

Following a motor vehicle accident (MVA), a client has sustained a transection spinal cord injury at L1. Which of the following conditions would the nurse expect to see the client in?

(A) The client will have to remain on a ventilator for life.
(B) The client is able to rotate the neck, but all limbs are paralyzed.
(C) The client has lost function on the entire left side of the body.
(D) The client has maintained use of his trunk and upper body, but both legs are paralyzed.

(B) Hemiplegia is paralysis on one side of the body. This client has right-sided hemiplegia. When transferring a client with hemiplegia, the wheelchair is placed parallel to the bed on the client's unaffected side. Once standing, the client can pivot the body around until the back is facing the chair and then reach for the far side of the chair with the unaffected arm. Placing the wheelchair perpendicular to the bed increases the distance the client has to pivot in order to sit in the chair. If the chair is placed on the affected side, the client will not be able to use the strong limbs as effectively. The wheelchair wheels should be locked for stability, and the nurse should brace the client from the front to assist with balance control.

(D) An L1 spinal cord injury is an injury at the first pair of lumbar nerves, which is located just below the waist. A transection spinal cord injury causes the areas of the body below the level of injury to be paralyzed. This client is most likely paralyzed from the waist down. Clients with this injury usually maintain body function of the trunk and upper body. Respiratory function is controlled by the thoracic spinal nerves (T1 to T12). With an injury in the lumbar spinal region, the client should have upper extremity function. The loss of function to one side of the body suggests that the injury did not penetrate the entire spinal cord.

Q-263

A client with Cushing's disease is hospitalized due to complications. The client is unconscious and being monitored for increased intracranial pressure (ICP). The LPN/LVN enters the room and finds the client decorticate posturing. Which of the following are manifestations of this phenomenon?

(A) Adducted, flexed upper extremities
(B) Outward rotation of the upper extremities
(C) Outward rotation of the lower extremities
(D) Extended upper extremities

Safe and Effective Care Environment:
Coordinated Care

Q-264

The LPN/LVN has just received report for the upcoming shift and plans to visit which client first?

(A) A client with pleurisy who is complaining of chest pain
(B) A client with pneumonia who has a temperature of $101.5°$F
(C) A client with chronic obstructive pulmonary disease (COPD) with a peripheral oxygen saturation of 89%
(D) A client with influenza who is complaining of shortness of breath

(A) Decorticate posturing is a sign of progressing neurological impairment. Manifestations include adduction and flexion of the upper extremities along with internal rotation of the lower extremities. Another type of posturing that is seen with progressing neurological impairment is decerabrate posturing. This involves extension and outward rotation of the upper extremities. Both types of posturing involve plantar flexion of the feet.

(D) The nurse must first assess any client with a condition that could be considered life threatening. A client with influenza who is experiencing shortness of breath needs to be assessed immediately to determine the problem. Chest pain is expected in a client with pleurisy, as is fever in a client with pneumonia. A client with COPD may have a lower than normal oxygen saturation and would be seen after the client with shortness of breath.

Physiological Integrity:
Physiological Adaptation

Q–265

Eight-year-old Joey was hit in the head with a baseball during Little League practice. His mother brings him to the emergency room. The magnetic resonance imaging (MRI) performed on the child's head shows a contusion. Joey is admitted to the hospital to be monitored. When asked by the mother, the LPN/LVN would correctly describe this condition as:

(A) Temporary loss of neurological function with no apparent tissue damage
(B) Bruising to the tissue of the brain
(C) Loss of brain function as a result of obstructed blood supply to a part of the brain
(D) Fracture to the skull bone

Physiological Integrity:
Physiological Adaptation

Q–266

A client with Raynaud's disease is experiencing symptoms of the disorder and visits the clinic. Which of the following statements from the client most likely indicates what caused exacerbation of these symptoms?

(A) "I just got back last night from a ski trip with my friends."
(B) "I've been in Africa for the past two weeks."
(C) "I just spent a week on the beaches of the Bahamas."
(D) "We sure have been getting a lot of rain around here lately."

A–265

(B) A contusion is a serious condition in which the tissue of the brain suffers bruising with possible surface bleeding. Answer (B) is correct. A cerebral concussion involves a temporary loss of neurological function following a head injury. Structural damage to the brain tissue does not occur with a concussion. Loss of brain function that results from a disruption to the supply of blood to a part of the brain is called a cerebrovascular accident (CVA) or stroke. A contusion is not defined as and does not necessarily involve a fracture to the skull bone.

A–266

(A) Raynaud's disease is a condition caused by irregular intervals of arteriolar vasoconstriction. Exacerbation of the symptoms of this disease are most commonly caused by exposure to cold climates. Emotional factors are also known to contribute to Raynaud's symptoms. Symptoms include coldness, pain, and pallor of the fingers or toes. The correct answer is (A). A recent ski trip indicates extended exposure to cold weather. Exposure to hot climates, sunny climates, and rainy climates do not contribute to these symptoms.

Q–267

The LPN/LVN is providing instruction to a client recently diagnosed with Raynaud's disease. Which of the following is recommended that clients with this condition avoid?

(A) Running
(B) Drinking alcoholic beverages
(C) Smoking
(D) Swimming

Q–268

Mr. Sandstone presents to the clinic after days of fatigue and lethargy. After blood tests are performed, the physician tells the client that he is experiencing anemia secondary to peptic ulcer disease (PUD). Mr. Sandstone's laboratory findings showed a decreased amount of which of the following in the blood?

(A) Leukocytes
(B) Platelets
(C) Reticulocytes
(D) Erythrocytes

Answers

(C) Raynaud's disease is a condition caused by random and sudden vasoconstriction. Therefore, it is advised that clients with Raynaud's disease avoid stimuli that cause vasoconstriction, including smoking. Running and other forms of exercise increase blood flow and promote vasodilatation. Drinking alcoholic beverages causes vasodilatation. Swimming is another form of exercise that promotes circulation.

(D) Anemia is the condition in which the number of red blood cells, or erythrocytes in the blood is low, answer (D). Leukocytes, or white blood cells, elevate during infection. A low leukocyte count indicates neutropenia, and the client's ability to fight infection is compromised. Reticulocytes are immature red blood cells. The reticulocyte count should rise during anemia as the bone marrow attempts to accommodate for the lost erythrocytes. A low platelet count might be present in clients with blood-clotting abnormalities.

Q–269

Which of the following is the best recommendation for a client with anemia to help reduce lethargy and fatigue?

(A) Take frequent resting periods.
(B) Take short walks twice a day.
(C) Eat a balanced diet using the food guide pyramid.
(D) Make sure to sleep for at least eight hours every night.

Safe and Effective Care Environment:
Coordinated Care

Q–270

The nurse is caring for four clients who have diabetes mellitus. At the beginning of the shift, which client should the nurse see first?

(A) A 58-year-old client with type 2 diabetes mellitus and a blood sugar level of 220 mg/dL
(B) A 17-year-old client with type 1 diabetes mellitus and a blood sugar level of 43 mg/dL
(C) A 7-year-old client with type 1 diabetes mellitus and a blood sugar level of 99 mg/dL
(D) A 75-year-old client with type 2 diabetes mellitus and a blood sugar level of 175 mg/dL

A-269

(A) Clients suffering from anemia will most likely experience a low level of energy. Although exercising, proper diet, and adequate sleep all help promote health and provide energy, allowing frequent periods for resting helps to balance activity and rest. This promotes maintenance of a consistent energy level throughout the day. The correct answer is (A).

A-270

(B) It is most important to attend to the client with hypoglycemia first because its onset is rapid and it can progress to unconsciousness and seizures shortly after the onset of symptoms. A client with a blood sugar that is elevated can tolerate it much longer than the client with hypoglycemia, and a blood sugar of 99 mg/dL is within the normal range.

Health Promotion and Maintenance

Q–271

Cancer is the second leading cause of death in the United States. Multiple etiological factors of cancer have been identified. Of the following, which have been found to lead to the development of some form of cancer? (Select all that apply.)

(A) Pathogenic microbes
(B) Dietary factors
(C) Pregnancy
(D) Oral contraceptive use
(E) Genetics
(F) Weight

Physiological Integrity:
Physiological Adaptation

Q–272

When a tumor is located at a body site, diagnostic evaluation involves staging of the size and extent of metastasis of the malignancy. Which of the following is NOT included in the system for this stage classification of tumors?

(A) N subclass
(B) M subclass
(C) T subclass
(D) G subclass

Answers

(A), **(B)**, **(D)**, **(E)**, and **(F)** are all correct. Certain pathogenic microbes have been identified as etiological factors to particular cancers. For example, infection with human papillomavirus (HPV) can lead to the development of cervical cancer. Studies have also shown that dietary factors, such as certain vitamin deficiencies or ingestion of carcinogens lead to certain forms of cancer. Oral contraceptive use has been found to contribute to cancers of the liver, breast, and female reproductive organs. Genetics and weight are also known etiological factors of various forms of cancer. The only incorrect answer is (C). Due to the hormones released during gestation, pregnancy has been shown to decrease the incidence of cancer.

(D) G subclass refers to grading, which is the classification of the cells of a tumor. This is the correct answer. The TNM classification system is the most commonly used system for evaluating tumor size and the existence and/or extent of metastasis of the cancer. The T represents classification of the original tumor. The N signifies existence and/or extent of lymph node involvement. The M refers to the existence and/or extent of metastasis.

Physiological Integrity:
Physiological Adaptation

Q–273

A hospitalized client begins to develop disseminated intravascular coagulopathy (DIC). Which of the following is an inaccurate statement regarding DIC?

(A) DIC is a sign of an underlying disease process.
(B) In DIC, coagulation time increases.
(C) Platelet count is low in DIC.
(D) Mortality rate for DIC exceeds 80%.

Physiological Integrity:
Physiological Adaptation

Q–274

The LPN/LVN stops at the side of the road after observing a motor vehicle accident (MVA). A young man is found lying on the ground outside of the car. The nurse observes that this man has a flail chest. Which of the following conditions would the nurse have identified to suggest this condition?

(A) Bulging of one side of the chest during expiration
(B) Tracheal shift to one side
(C) Subcutaneous emphysema
(D) Central cyanosis

Answers

(B) Disseminated intravascular coagulopathy (DIC) is not a disease itself, but a sign that a serious underlying disease process is occurring. Body mechanisms that maintain proper circulation are severely malfunctioning. This causes tiny clots to form throughout the body, while at the same time coagulation time is shortened. Fibrinogen levels and platelet counts are low. If the underlying cause is not identified and corrected, DIC is seriously life threatening. The underlying disease process is not found or stopped in more than 80% of those who develop this condition, leading to death.

(A) Flail chest occurs when multiple rib fractures have occurred causing segments of the rib bone to float in the rib cage. The rib segment is sucked inward with inhalation causing an area of the chest to depress. With expiration, this area of the chest will bulge as it is blown outward, answer (A). Tracheal shift is a manifestation of a tension pneumothorax as air becomes trapped in the pleural space. Subcutaneous emphysema occurs when air escapes into the skin tissue. Although it does not suggest flail chest, subcutaneous emphysema can occur in any type of injury to the pulmonary structures. Bluish discoloration of the mucous membranes of the mouth is called central cyanosis. This is a symptom of pneumothorax.

Q–275

The LPN/LVN is reviewing a client's medical record. On the physician's progress notes the nurse sees "PERRLA." Which of the following cranial nerves is not associated with this abbreviation?

(A) Cranial nerve IV
(B) Cranial nerve VI
(C) Cranial nerve II
(D) Cranial nerve III

Q–276

The LPN/LVN is assessing a postoperative client following abdominal surgery. The nurse notes that there is an excessive amount of drainage from the client's Salem sump tube. Which of the following would the nurse monitor the client for?

(A) Respiratory acidosis
(B) Respiratory alkalosis
(C) Metabolic acidosis
(D) Metabolic alkalosis

Answers

(C) "PERRLA" stands for "pupils are equal, round, and reactive to light and accommodation." These assessments indicate motor function to the eye. Cranial nerves III (Oculomotor), IV (Trochlear), and VI (Abducens) are responsible for movements of the eye muscles, including the pupils. Cranial nerve II (the Optic nerve) is responsible for visual acuity. Answer (C) is the appropriate choice.

(D) Salem sump is a type of nasogastric tube used commonly following abdominal surgery to remove fluid and gas from the upper gastrointestinal (GI) tract to allow healing to occur. The GI tract is primarily responsible for maintaining metabolic acid-base balance. The fluid contents removed by this tube will contain hydrochloric acid. The removal of an excessive amount of this acid can lead to a disturbance in the acid-base balance in the body. There is less acid and more base in the body, which leads to alkalosis. The correct answer is (D). This situation could lead to metabolic alkalosis. Respiratory acidosis and respiratory alkalosis are caused by breathing difficulties.

Physiological Integrity:
Basic Care and Comfort

Q–277

A newborn with cleft palate is scheduled for operative correction of the defect. Prior to the operation, the child is showing signs of growth failure. Which of the following manifestations is most likely a contributing factor to this condition caused by the defect?

(A) Sucking difficulties
(B) Inability to properly digest
(C) Frequent regurgitation
(D) Constipation

Physiological Integrity:
Physiological Adaptation

Q–278

A newborn is delivered with bilateral clubfoot (talipes equinovarus or TEV). Which of the following indicates that surgical intervention is needed?

(A) Heels of the feet are pulled in and the toes point inward.
(B) Heels of the casted feet are turned out and the toes point outward.
(C) Failure of the deformity to respond to serial casting.
(D) The feet have undergone manipulation and casting for eight consecutive weeks.

Answers

(**A**) Cleft palate is a congenital defect that is caused by an incomplete fusion during embryonic development of the palate in the roof of the mouth. This defect may only involve the soft palate or may extend through the hard palate, leaving an opening from the mouth into the nose. Prior to surgical repair, feeding a newborn with cleft palate can be very difficult due to decreased sucking ability and escape of food from the nose. Unless other defects are present, digestion is normal once the food passes the oral cavity. Frequent regurgitation and constipation are not known to be caused by cleft palates in newborns.

(**C**) Clubfoot (talipes equinovarus) is a deformity of one or both feet where the heels are turned in and the toes point inward. The cause is not always known, but other congenital defects can contribute. Breech position or overcrowding in utero may also be a causative factor. Serial casting, manipulation, and casting repeated every 1 to 2 weeks for 8 to 12 weeks is begun very soon after the deformity is noticed at birth. The casts are applied with the heels of the feet turned out and the toes pointed inward to stretch the muscles appropriately. If the deformity fails to correct after serial casting, surgical intervention is necessary.

Health Promotion and Maintenance

Q–279

The mother of a 22-month-old toddler who has suffered from frequent otitis media (OM) infections asks the nurse what could cause these ear infections to reoccur so often. Select all of the following that are normal characteristics of young children that predispose them to development of otitis media.

(A) Narrow eustachian tubes
(B) Undeveloped cartilage lining the ear
(C) Short eustachian tubes
(D) Formula or breast milk used as primary nutrition
(E) Normal positioning of young children
(F) Hormonal defense responses of young children

Physiological Integrity:
Basic Care and Comfort

Q–280

An infant is receiving digoxin (Lanoxin) for a congenital heart defect. Which of the following interventions by the nurse will also decrease the workload of the heart?

(A) Scheduling the parents to visit for short periods of time at arranged intervals
(B) Organizing nursing care to allow long rest periods for the infant
(C) Providing smaller feedings at frequent intervals
(D) Providing feedings through a nasogastric tube

Answers

(B), (C), (E), and (F) are all correct answers. Otitis media (OM), inflammation of the middle ear, is a very common disease of early childhood. Factors that predispose young children to frequent otitis media infections include: short, wide, straight eustachian tubes; horizontal lie of the eustachian tube; undeveloped cartilage lining of the eustachian tube; immature hormonal defenses; and frequent lying position of infants and toddlers. All of these are factors that are normal to the immature anatomy and physiology of young children. Young children do not have narrow eustachian tubes. Due to their underdeveloped digestive systems, formula and/or breast milk is necessary for primary nutrition of very young children.

(B) Allowing the infant long rest periods decreases energy demands, which decreases how hard the heart needs to work to circulate oxygen to tissues and organs through the blood supply. Organizing nursing care to allow quiet and undisturbed time intervals for the infant will accomplish this. The correct answer is (B). The parents should not be discouraged from visiting at any time to promote parent-infant bonding. Feeding at frequent intervals decreases the time the infant can rest, which increases energy demands of the body. Nasogastric feedings would be used only if the child has increased energy demands caused by prolonged feeding times or a poor sucking reflex.

Q–281

The LPN/LVN is responsible for continually observing clients for clinical features that suggest the need for medical evaluation. Which of the following children is displaying signs of hypertrophic pyloric stenosis (HPS)?

(A) A child with diarrhea and a poor appetite
(B) A toddler who cries with abdominal palpation
(C) A child with stool that tests positive for blood
(D) An infant who vomits after feedings

Q–282

A child with a few vesicular skin lesions on her face is brought to the emergency room. She is diagnosed with chickenpox. To prevent transmission of chickenpox through direct contact, the LPN/LVN initiates contact precautions. Which of the following should *also* be initiated to isolate this illness?

(A) Reverse isolation
(B) Airborne precautions
(C) Standard precautions
(D) Droplet precautions

A-281

(D) Hypertrophic pyloric stenosis (HPS) is a condition that involves thickening of the muscle surrounding the pyloric sphincter area of the gastrointestinal tract. The muscular hypertrophy leads to inability for the stomach contents to empty into the small intestines, which leads to vomiting after meals and failure to gain weight, answer (D). Diarrhea, anorexia with weight loss, and occasional vomiting are classic signs of ileocolic intussusception. Pain with abdominal palpation and blood in the stool are not known to be associated with HPS.

A-282

(B) Airborne precautions are used to prevent transmission of microbes that are found in droplets that are smaller than 5 microns. Along with direct contact, chickenpox is also transmitted in airborne droplets smaller than 5 microns. Reverse isolation involves precautions that inhibit transmission of microbes to imunosuppressed clients, including burn victims and clients receiving chemotherapy. Standard precautions are used to care for all hospitalized clients regardless of their diagnosis. Droplet precautions are used for clients with known or suspected illnesses transmitted by larger particle droplets (more than 5 microns).

Q–283

The parents of a child with sickle cell anemia (SCA) ask the LPN/LVN how their child could have this illness if neither of them has it. Which of the following is NOT an accurate statement regarding the genetics of this disease?

(A) "Both of you are carriers of the sickle cell trait."
(B) "Although you are unaffected, all of the children you have together will have a 1 in 4 chance of having the illness."
(C) "At least one of you is a carrier of the sickle cell trait."
(D) "Any children you have together that do not have the illness have a 2 in 3 chance of being carriers."

Physiological Integrity:
Physiological Adaptation

Q–284

A child is admitted to the hospital with respiratory difficulty and failure to thrive. Diagnostic tests indicate the child has cystic fibrosis. Which of the following comments from the child's mother supports this diagnosis?

(A) The mother states, this child "seems to require more sleep than [her] other children."
(B) The mother says, "I notice a salty taste when I kiss my child."
(C) The mother states that her child appears to bruise easily.
(D) The mother says her child doesn't cry very often.

A–283

(C) The gene for sickle cell anemia is autosomal recessive. This means that both parents of clients with sickle cell anemia are carriers of the trait for the illness but are unaffected by the illness themselves. Any children of two carriers of the trait have a 1 in 4 chance of being affected by the illness. Any children of this couple who do not have sickle cell anemia have a 2 in 3 chance of carrying the trait for the illness. Answer (C) is the correct choice. Both parents of a child with this illness must be carriers.

A–284

(B) Due to high amounts of salt production, parents of children with cystic fibrosis often comment that they notice a salty taste when they kiss their child/children. The salt is secreted in tears, saliva, and perspiration. The correct answer is (B). Sweat chloride tests are used to diagnose cystic fibrosis. Diagnosis is indicated if this test is positive and the child either has symptoms associated with the illness or genetic predisposition. Sleep is essential for growth and development, and patterns of sleep differ among children. Easy bruising and infrequent crying are not symptoms associated with cystic fibrosis.

Health Promotion and Maintenance

Q–285

What is the best site for assessing the heart rate of a three-year-old child?

Safe and Effective Care Environment:
Safety and Infection Control

Q–286

Mrs. Emmit brings her three-year-old son to the emergency department after discovering that the child has ingested an unknown amount of multi-vitamins with iron. After treatment is provided, the mother and child are being sent home. Which of the following are appropriate teaching points for prevention of ingestion of toxic substances? (Select all that apply.)

(A) Have someone watching the child at all times.
(B) Discard any potentially poisonous materials that are in the home.
(C) Keep toxic substances in locked compartments.
(D) Clearly label all medicines.
(E) Be cautious of placing live plants within the child's reach.

A-285

ANSWER: Apical site

RATIONALE: Under the age of five, the best way for assessing the heart rate is by auscultating the apical pulse. It is more difficult to palpate an accurate heart rate at other sites on young children because of the speed of the pulse and constitution of body tissues. The carotid or brachial sites are often palpated during cardiopulmonary resuscitation (CPR).

A-286

(C), **(D)**, and **(E)** are all correct answers. Keeping a constant eye on children and discarding all poisonous materials from the home is unrealistic. However, excessive amounts of poisonous materials should not be stored in the home. Potentially poisonous substances should not only be placed out of reach but also locked in a compartment to prevent child access. Medications and pills should be appropriately labeled and in childproof containers. Some plants are poisonous if ingested. Keeping live plants hung or otherwise out of children's reach is a good general rule. Otherwise, knowing which plants are poisonous and avoiding placing them in the house should be advised.

Physiological Integrity:
Reduction of Risk Potential

Q–287

A five-year-old girl is brought to the emergency department complaining of a sore throat and pain when swallowing. She has uncontrolled drooling and a temperature of 102.4° F. The physician orders a throat culture for diagnosis. Which of the following is the most appropriate nursing action at this time?

(A) Obtain the culture by swabbing the oropharynx and tonsillar regions of the throat.
(B) Allow the child to sit on her mother's lap while obtaining the culture.
(C) Have the child sit straight up, open the mouth, extend the tongue, and say "ah" to swab the throat.
(D) Question the physician's order.

Physiological Integrity:
Reduction of Risk Potential

Q–288

The LPN/LVN is caring for a seven-year-old boy with leukemia. When assessing routine vital signs, which route is contraindicated for obtaining the body temperature of a child with leukemia?

(A) Oral
(B) Axillary
(C) Rectal
(D) Tympanic

Answers

(D) Severe sore throat with dysphagia (difficulty swallowing), drooling, and high fever are all suggestive that the child has epiglotittis, which is a form of croup. Other symptoms include stridor, orthopnea, rapid pulse, and rapid respirations. Inserting objects into the back of the throat can precipitate obstruction of the airway by causing further tissue inflammation. The nurse should question the physician's order, answer (D). All other answers would be appropriate if obtaining a throat culture was not contraindicated.

(C) Leukemia patients have a decreased ability to fight infection. All routes for obtaining body temperature are appropriate except rectal. This is due to potential complications caused by inserting a probe into the rectum. Perirectal tissue is very susceptible to becoming abscessed if the skin is broken.

Health Promotion and Maintenance

Q-289

An eight-year-old boy diagnosed with leukemia is scheduled for a bone marrow aspiration. Prior to the procedure, the child is uncooperative and anxious. Which of the following is the most appropriate intervention by the nurse for this child?

(A) Acknowledge the child's fear and explain to the child that this is a rather simple and quick procedure.
(B) Allow the child to play with a model of a bone after using it to explain the procedure in usual medical terms.
(C) Ask the parents to calm the child.
(D) Tell the child that if his behavior continues the doctors will be very upset with him.

Physiological Integrity:
Reduction of Risk Potential

Q-290

The Hirschberg test is performed on a $2\frac{1}{2}$-year-old child to check eye alignment. Which of the following abnormalities is this testing for?

(A) Strabismus
(B) Hypertelorism
(C) Amblyopia
(D) Papilledema

A–289

(**B**) Anxiety prior to a procedure can be relieved by informing the child of what they will encounter. Invalid assumptions are often made that children know more about their bodies than they do. Allowing a child to play with and manipulate models, dolls, or equipment will help the child feel more comfortable with the situation, answer (B). Explaining the procedure as simple and quick is not necessarily accurate and will probably not ease the child's anxiety. Asking the parents to control the child's reactions or attempting to manipulate the child with reward, punishment, or threat is inappropriate in dealing with this anxiety.

A–290

(**A**) Alignment of the eyes is tested to detect nonbinocular vision, or strabismus. In strabismus, also known as cross eye, one eye deviates from the point of fixation. This can lead to disuse of the eye and eventually blindness. This blindness is called amblyopia, which is blindness that is not caused by physical disease or defect. Hypertelorism is large spacing between the eyes. Papilledema is swelling of the optic nerve, which is often an indication of increased intracranial pressure.

Safe and Effective Care Environment:
Coordinated Care

Q–291

A male teenager with Type 1 diabetes mellitus suddenly complains that he is "shaky and dizzy." His respirations are shallow, and he is having difficulty speaking. Which of the following is the nursing action of highest priority?

(A) Administer dextrose 50% intravenously.
(B) Have him drink a glass of orange juice.
(C) Give 15 units of regular insulin.
(D) Test the glucose level of a capillary blood sample.

Physiological Integrity:
Pharmacological Therapies

Q–292

A 14-year-old girl recently diagnosed with Type 1 diabetes mellitus is receiving instruction regarding self-injection techniques. The LPN/LVN would inform the client that onset of action varies among injection sites. Arrange the following injection sites in the correct order, starting with the site that absorbs solution the fastest.

(A) Arm
(B) Abdomen
(C) Buttock
(D) Leg

Answers

(B) The teenager is exhibiting signs of hypoglycemia. Since he is alert and able to swallow, he should immediately ingest a source of concentrated sugar, such as orange juice, to raise the blood sugar, answer (B). Intravenous administration of a sugar substance is reserved for clients in an unconscious state or who are unable to ingest food or drink. Giving insulin at this time would contribute to further hypoglycemia, which is fatal to the client. Testing the capillary blood glucose level is not the highest priority intervention at this time.

(B), **(A)**, **(D)**, and **(C)**. The abdomen is the injection site that has the fastest absorption rate. Injections at this site become effective in a very short period of time. Injections in the arm are absorbed slightly slower than in the abdomen. The absorption rate in the leg is slow, followed by the buttock, which has the slowest absorption rate. Clients are advised to use one site for four to six injections and then move to another site. Knowing absorption rate of the various sites is important for planning interventions related to management of diabetes mellitus.

Questions

Physiological Integrity:
Reduction of Risk Potential

Q–293

Immediately following an open appendectomy, a 16-year-old client is anxious to return to school and extracurricular activities. The LPN/LVN informs the client that if her recovery is normal and without complications, she should be able to return to school in what time period?

(A) 1 to 2 weeks
(B) 2 to 3 weeks
(C) 3 to 4 weeks
(D) 6 weeks

Safe and Effective Care Environment:
Safety and Infection Control

Q–294

When should the LPN/LVN perform hand hygiene with soap and water instead of alcohol-based hand cleaner? Select all that apply.

(A) After removing gloves
(B) Before eating food
(C) After touching nasal secretions
(D) After administering an intramuscular injection
(E) After using the toilet

Answers

A–293

(A) Following an uncomplicated open appendectomy and recovery, the teenager should be able to return to school in one to two weeks, answer **(A)**. It is advised for strenuous activity to be avoided until healing is complete, which may take one to two additional weeks. It is unnecessary to keep an adolescent out of school for more than two weeks unless complications have inhibited healing or caused a worsened condition.

A–294

(B), **(C)**, and **(E)** The most important times for the nurse to perform hand washing are before eating, after using the toilet, and after coming in contact with nasal secretions. Using alcohol-based hand cleanser would be appropriate after removing gloves and after administering an IM injection.

Physiological Integrity:
Pharmacological Therapies

Q–295

The physician has ordered Tylenol 15 mg/kg p.o. every 4 to 6 hours for a 76-lb child. According to this order, what is the maximum amount in milligrams that the LPN/LVN can administer in a single dose?

(A) 15 mg
(B) 518 mg
(C) 1140 mg
(D) 2508 mg

Safe and Effective Care Environment:
Safety and Infection Control

Q–296

The LPN/LVN visits the home of a family with an 18-month-old child for a safety inspection. Which of the following would alert the nurse to provide further childhood safety instructions?

(A) The water heater is set to 120° F.
(B) All electrical outlets are covered.
(C) The child is eating frozen grapes at lunch time.
(D) The child plays with play dough.

Answers

(B) The first step to solve this problem is to convert pounds to kilograms by dividing the weight in pounds by 2.2 (2.2 lbs = 1 kg):

$$\frac{76 \text{ lb}}{2.2} = 34.5 \text{ kg}$$

Next, multiply weight in kilograms by allowed dosage in milligrams per kilogram:

34.5 kg × 15 mg/kg = 517.5

Rounded off to the nearest whole number, the correct answer is 518, answer (B).

(C) Whole grapes given to a child of this age pose the threat of choking. To prevent choking, parents should avoid allowing the child to eat whole, round foods or hard foods, such as vegetable sticks, which can get caught in a child's airway. Setting the water heater to 120° F or below, covering electrical outlets with proper coverings, and allowing the child to play with play dough are all appropriate in the environment of a child of this age.

Q–297

A 12-year-old female is brought to the clinic by her mother because she is complaining of extremely painful cramping with menstruation. Which of the following could be recommended to relieve symptoms of dysmenorrhea?

(A) "Taking cool showers and swimming activities may help ease the pain you are experiencing."
(B) "Taking Vitamin E and Vitamin B_6 supplements have been found to help decrease these symptoms."
(C) "Too much activity can worsen the symptoms of dysmenorrhea."
(D) "Be sure to consume plenty of sodium in your diet."

Physiological Integrity:
Pharmacological Therapies

Q–298

A client visits the clinic to get information on birth control methods. The nurse reviews the client's medical history before she is seen by the physician. Which of the following contraindicates prescribing oral contraceptives to this client?

(A) History of thrombophlebitis
(B) History of migraines
(C) History of spontaneous abortion
(D) History of dysmenorrhea

Answers

A-297

(B) The primary cause of dysmenorrhea is production of high concentrations of prostaglandins. Vitamin E is a mild prostaglandin inhibitor, which may help ease the painful symptoms associated with menstruation. Vitamin B_6 helps decrease other symptoms such as bloating and irritability. Answer (B) is correct. Other actions that are helpful to decrease symptoms of dysmenorrhea include taking a warm bath, sipping herbal tea, or using a heating pad to soothe and increase blood flow. Daily exercise, especially aerobic exercise helps diminish cramping and other menstrual symptoms. Avoiding salt can help decrease bloating and fluid retention during menstruation.

A-298

(A) Oral contraceptives are a commonly used method of birth control. These medications contain particular dosages of hormones, particularly estrogen and progestin. Use of oral contraceptives is contraindicated for clients with a history of thrombophlebitis or thromboembolic disease due to associated risk of thrombus formation. Oral contraceptives can increase frequency and severity of migraines. Use is not contraindicated, but frequent monitoring is advised for these clients. Clients with a history of spontaneous abortion (more commonly known as miscarriage) may use oral contraceptives. Oral contraceptives are often used to ease symptoms of dysmenorrhea.

Q–299

A couple visits the clinic after deciding they do not want to have any more children. While reviewing the options for sterilization, the couple is advised of all advantages and disadvantages associated with each method, including the complications of the various procedures. Which of the following is NOT a common complication associated with the procedure for tubal ligation?

(A) Perforation of the bowel
(B) Injury to abdominal tissue
(C) Infection
(D) Early menopause

Q–300

A client suspects that she is pregnant and visits the clinic. Of the following changes caused by pregnancy, which is the only positive sign that the client is pregnant?

(A) Enlarged abdomen
(B) Positive pregnancy tests
(C) Detection of fetal heartbeat
(D) Uterine contractions

A–299

(D) Tubal ligation is a surgical method for female sterilization, which involves obstructing the fallopian tubes. Complications commonly caused by this procedure include coagulation burns to bowel or other abdominal tissue, bowel perforation, pain, infection, hemorrhage, and adverse effects of anesthesia. This does not involve removal of hormone-producing organs. Therefore, early menopause is not caused by this procedure. Answer (D) is the correct choice.

A–300

(C) Positive signs of pregnancy are detected changes that provide objective, conclusive proof of pregnancy. Detection of fetal heart rate, fetal movement palpated by a professional, and visualization of the fetus usually by sonography are the only positive signs of pregnancy. Answer (C) is correct. Enlarged abdomen, positive pregnancy tests, and uterine contractions are only probable signs of pregnancy.

Health Promotion and Maintenance

Q–301

Following are the cardinal movements of the fetus during labor. Arrange the answer choices in the order, from first to last, in which they occur.

(A) Extension and restitution
(B) Internal rotation
(C) External rotation
(D) Descent
(E) Expulsion
(F) Flexion

Health Promotion and Maintenance

Q–302

Many terms are used to describe the progression of labor. Which of the following is a correct explanation of the term "station"?

(A) The location of the presenting part in relationship to the ischial spines
(B) The point at which the largest diameter of the presenting part reaches or passes through the pelvic inlet
(C) The movement of the cervical muscle up into the side walls of the uterus
(D) Tightening and shortening of the uterus during labor

Answers

(D), **(F)**, **(B)**, **(A)**, **(C)**, **(E)** is the correct order. Descent is the movement in which the fetus moves into the pelvic inlet. Flexion occurs as the head of the fetus meets resistance against the soft tissues and musculature of the pelvis. Internal rotation is the movement that the fetal head must make in order to fit the diameter of the pelvic cavity. Extension occurs as the fetal head passes under the symphysis pubis. Restitution is the turning of the fetal head to align with the back of the fetus after it is free of pelvic resistance. During external rotation the shoulders rotate opposite to the rotation of the head to allow for the final cardinal movement, expulsion of the fetal body.

(A) Station is defined as the location of the presenting part in relationship to the ischial spines, which is declared using numbers from −5 to +5. The point at which the largest diameter of the presenting part reaches or passes through the pelvic inlet is called engagement. Effacement is the movement of cervical muscle up into the side walls of the uterus. Uterine contractions involve tightening and shortening of the uterine muscle during labor.

Health Promotion and Maintenance

Q–303

A pregnant woman at full term is experiencing frequent contractions and comes to the hospital. After performing a pelvic exam, the physician tells the client that it appears the back of the head is descending first and is against the front right side of her pelvis. Which of the following fetal positions has the physician just described?

(A) LOA
(B) LOP
(C) ROA
(D) ROT

Health Promotion and Maintenance

Q–304

A laboring mother is completely dilated (10 cm) and 100% effaced. She has been pushing for about 20 minutes, and the fetal head is crowning. What stage of labor is this client in?

(A) First stage
(B) Second stage
(C) Third stage
(D) Fourth stage

Answers

(C) Three notations are used to describe fetal position. The first (right, "R" or left, "L") refers to the side of the maternal pelvis that the presenting part is facing. The second (occiput, "O", mentum, "M", sacrum, "S", or acromion process, "A") refers to the landmark of the body that is the presenting part. The third (anterior, "A", posterior, "P", or transverse, "T") refers to whether the presenting part is facing more towards the front, back, or side of the maternal pelvis. In this case, the back of the fetal head (occiput) is facing the right and front side of the maternal pelvis. Right, occiput, anterior (ROA), or answer (C), is correct.

(B) The first stage of labor is from the onset of true labor to when the cervix is completely dilated and effaced. The second stage of labor begins when the cervix is fully dilated and effaced and ends with the birth of the baby, answer (B). The second stage is when the mother pushes with contractions to assist movement of the fetus through the birth canal. The third stage of labor involves the expulsion of the placenta. The fourth stage of labor involves contractions of the uterus to control bleeding and decrease uterine muscle size.

Health Promotion and Maintenance

Q–305

A laboring client is 7 cm dilated. She states that she has an incredible urge to push with each contraction. Which of the following statements by the LPN/LVN is accurate?

(A) "You can begin pushing with the next contraction."
(B) "You may deliver the baby without the physician present if you start pushing now."
(C) "Pushing at this time may prolong your labor."
(D) "You may need to move your bowels. I will get the bedpan."

Health Promotion and Maintenance

Q–306

A pregnant woman at full term should be advised of signs that labor is about to begin. Which of the following are premonitory signs, which indicate impending true labor?

(A) Increased frequency of contractions
(B) Lightening
(C) White vaginal discharge
(D) Fatigue
(E) Bloody show
(F) Spontaneous rupture of membranes

Answers

A–305

(C) Pushing before the cervix is completely dilated may inhibit progression of labor. The presenting part of the fetus compresses the partially dilated cervix, causing it to swell and enlarge. The correct answer is (C). The nurse should encourage breathing techniques and focus to distract the laboring client from the urge to push. Telling the client that she can push at this time is inappropriate. Telling the client that delivery may occur without the physician present is inaccurate and inappropriate for this situation. The urge is more likely due to pressure of the fetal head against the pelvis than a need for the client to move her bowels.

A–306

(A), **(B)**, **(E)**, and **(F)** are the correct answers. Premonitory signs of labor include: Braxton Hicks contractions, which are irregular, and intermittent contractions, which occur throughout pregnancy and become more frequent as true labor approaches; lightening or settling of the fetus into the pelvic inlet; pink-tinged secretions called bloody show that indicate the mucous plug has been expelled; and spontaneous rupture of the amniotic sac called the "membranes." Fatigue is common throughout pregnancy. A pregnant woman often experiences a sudden burst of energy just prior to true labor. White vaginal discharge is common throughout pregnancy and does not indicate that labor is near.

Health Promotion and Maintenance

Q-307

It is often difficult for a pregnant client to determine if she is actually in labor or experiencing false symptoms. Which of the following is an accurate difference between true and false labor?

(A) In false labor, walking intensifies contractions. In true labor, walking eases contractions.

(B) Discomfort of false labor is felt mostly in the back. Discomfort of true labor is felt in the abdomen.

(C) Contractions of both true and false labor progressively increase in intensity.

(D) Intervals between true labor contractions shorten progressively. Intervals in false labor are irregular or produce no change.

Safe and Effective Care Environment:
Safety and Infection Control

Q-308

The nurse has received notice that a client with a contagious illness who will need airborne precautions will be admitted to the unit. The nurse knows that this client may have which communicable disease? Select all that apply.

(A) Chickenpox
(B) Rubeola
(C) Rubella
(D) Tuberculosis
(E) Influenza

Answers

A–307

(D) Walking intensifies contraction discomfort in true labor and either produces no effect or eases contraction discomfort in false labor. False labor discomfort is felt in the abdomen. The discomfort of true labor usually begins in the back and radiates to the front. Contractions of true labor increase in intensity while the intensity of false labor contractions usually remains constant. True labor can be identified when the intervals between contractions progressively shorten. False labor contractions can be very irregular or remain the same distance apart.

A–308

(A), **(B)**, and **(D)** Communicable diseases that are classified as airborne are tuberculosis, chicken pox, and rubeola. Influenza, rubella, and both streptococcal and meningococcal meningitis are transmitted by droplet.

Q–309

Which of the following interventions should be performed to prevent the most common complication associated with treatment of pain during labor using an epidural block?

(A) Preloading a rapid infusion of intravenous fluids
(B) Assessing the sensation level on the client's body during continuous epidural administration
(C) Intermittent urinary catheterizations
(D) Blood pressure monitoring every 5 to 15 minutes

Q–310

Fetal heart rate is carefully monitored throughout pregnancy and during labor to assess fetal well-being. Which of the following represents an appropriate fetal heart rate?

(A) 108
(B) 127
(C) 170
(D) 185

Answers

(A) The most common complication associated with epidural block is hypotension. Preloading a rapid infusion of intravenous fluids is a common measure used to prevent this complication, answer (A). Frequent blood pressure is often taken to assess for hypotension. This method is for monitoring, and not a preventative measure. Assessing the point on the client's body that senses stimuli is important to avoid oversedation and to ensure effectiveness of the medication. This is unrelated to the most common complication, hypotension. Urinary retention is common complication, but it is not the most common complication of epidural use.

(B) The appropriate range for fetal heart rate is 120 to 160 beats per minute (BPM). Answer (B) is correct. Fetal tachycardia, heart rate above this range, can indicate a chronic cardiopulmonary dysfunction. Fetal bradycardia, heart rate below this range, can indicate an acute or immediate cardiopulmonary problem. Fetal heart rate outside of this range can also indicate hypoxia or congenital heart defects.

Health Promotion and Maintenance

Q–311

After treatment for infertility, a client becomes pregnant with triplets. With pregnancy of more than one fetus, incidence of complications increases. Select all of the following that are implications associated with multiple gestation.

(A) Increased risk of preterm labor
(B) Increased risk of infection
(C) Increased need for labor induction
(D) Increased risk of maternal death
(E) Babies born with lower birth weight

Health Promotion and Maintenance

Q–312

A client is pregnant with her third child. Medical history of the client indicates a previous precipitate labor and birth. Which of the following interventions would NOT be expected during the labor of the present pregnancy?

(A) Use of magnesium sulfate
(B) Close monitoring of the fetus for hypoxia
(C) The nurse stays at the bedside constantly or as much as possible.
(D) Amnioinfusion will be performed.

A–311

(A) and (E) are correct choices. Preterm labor and low-birth-weight babies often result from multiple birth pregnancies. Other dangers include increased risk for postpartum hemorrhage, increased risk for Cesarean birth, increased risk of prematurity of newborns, and increased risk for congenital anomalies. Infection rates, induction of labor, and maternal deaths are not manifestations known to increase with multiple gestation.

A–312

(D) A precipitate labor and birth is a rapid labor and birth that is completed within three hours. This can cause abruption of the placenta, extensive lacerations, and fetal or neonatal distress. The goal of the labor process for a client with this history is to slow contractions and labor as much as possible. Magnesium sulfate and tocolytic drugs such as terbutaline are often used to slow uterine contractions. The fetus is closely monitored for fetal distress, which includes hypoxia. Due to the intense situation and fast pace of a precipitate labor and birth, the nurse will stay at the bedside as much as possible during labor. Amnioinfusion is instillation of fluid into the amniotic sac within the uterus to treat oligohydramnios. This is not done to prevent precipitate labor and birth. Answer (D) is correct.

Psychosocial Integrity

Q–313

Shortly after a client finds out that her recently delivered fetus had died in utero, the nurse attempts to console the client and her partner. Which of the following is the most therapeutic action by the nurse at this time?

(A) The nurse says to the client, "You're still young, and you'll have many more pregnancies."
(B) The nurse brings the stillborn infant for the parents to see and hold.
(C) The nurse states, "At least it wasn't a 2-year-old that died."
(D) The nurse leaves the couple alone to grieve.

Health Promotion and Maintenance

Q–314

After experiencing vaginal bleeding, a 33-week-pregnant woman is brought to the emergency room by paramedics. Which of the following complications of pregnancy can vaginal bleeding indicate? (Select all that apply.)

(A) Hyperemesis gravidarum
(B) Preeclampsia
(C) Hydramnios
(D) Abruptio placentae
(E) Impending spontaneous abortion
(F) Placenta previa

Answers

(B) The comments in answers (A) and (C) are not therapeutic. The nurse is minimizing the situation instead of allowing the parents to express grief related to the experience. The nurse should offer her presence to the grieving couple as much as possible. Saying the "right thing" is not necessary. Just being with the couple provides comfort and prevents feelings of isolation. Answer (B) is the most appropriate. Offering a time to see and hold the stillborn infant is therapeutic to the parents. However, they should be prepared for what to expect the infant to look like.

(D), **(E)**, and **(F)** are the correct choices. Of the above choices, vaginal bleeding can indicate abruptio placentae, impending spontaneous abortion, or placenta previa. Abruptio placentae is the premature separation of the placenta from the uterine wall. Placenta previa involves improper implantation of the placenta into the lower section of the uterus. Hyperemesis gravidarum is excessive vomiting during pregnancy. Preeclampsia is characterized by hypertension, edema, and albuminuria. Hydramnios is an excess of amniotic fluid that causes overextension of the uterus. Hyperemesis gravidarum, preeclampsia, and hydramnios are not conditions that involve vaginal bleeding during pregnancy.

Health Promotion and Maintenance

Q–315

One minute after delivery, assessment findings of a newborn include a heart rate of 120 BPM, vigorous crying, some flexion of extremities, and bluish-colored arms and legs. Calculate the one-minute Apgar score of the neonate.

(A) 5
(B) 8
(C) 9
(D) 10

Health Promotion and Maintenance

Q–316

A client finds out at 22-weeks gestation that she is pregnant with twins. The client is anxious to discover if the twins are fraternal or identical. Which of the following is accurate pertaining to the occurrence of twins?

(A) Fraternal twins often share a single placenta.
(B) Identical twinning is caused by fertilization of two eggs.
(C) Twinning occurs in approximately 1 in 80 pregnancies.
(D) Congenital anomalies are more prominent in fraternal twins than identical twins.

Answers

(B) The Apgar scoring system is used to evaluate the physical condition of a newborn at birth and shortly after birth. This assessment is usually done at 1 minute and 5 minutes following birth. This system involves five criteria, each receiving a score from 0 to 2. These criteria include:

—Heart rate (absent = 0, below 100 BPM = 1, above 100 BPM = 2)
—Respiratory effort (absent = 0, slow or irregular = 1, good crying = 2)
—Muscle tone (flaccid = 0, some extremity flexion = 1, active motion = 2)
—Reflex irritability (none = 0, grimace = 1, vigorous cry = 2)
—Color (pale = 0, blue extremities = 1, completely pink = 2).

This infant would have a one-minute Apgar score of 8 out of 10, answer (B).

(C) Twinning, whether fraternal or identical, occurs in approximately 1 pregnancy of every 80, answer (C). Fraternal twins are the result of the fertilization of two eggs, each with its own placenta. Identical twinning is a random event that results from division of a single fertilized ovum during early embryonic development. Congenital anomalies are more common in identical twins than in fraternal twins. Survival rate is also lower for identical twins than fraternal twins.

Q–317

The LPN/LVN enters the room of a client at an inpatient psychiatric facility and overhears a conversation between the client and a lawyer. The client states that she is "experiencing client abuse and being held against her will." Which of the following does this conversation represent?

(A) Right to confidentiality
(B) Breach of telephone privileges of psychiatric inpatients
(C) Invasion of privacy
(D) Right to judicial involvement

Q–318

A 30-year-old male client is admitted to the psychiatric facility for observation and treatment of newly identified schizophrenia. Medications from which of the following classifications would most likely be prescribed as a part of this client's treatment?

(A) Antianxiety agents
(B) Hypnotics
(C) Antipsychotics
(D) Anticonvulsants

A–317

(A) Confidentiality awards the client the right to reveal information about care and treatment to others. The client has the right to discuss the situation with an attorney. In turn, the attorney is forbidden by law to disclose information without client consent, according to privileged communication. Invasion of privacy has not occurred since the nurse is directly involved in the client's care. Disclosure of this information to anyone not directly involved in the client's care would be considered breach of confidentiality. Judicial involvement is not a documented client right.

A–318

(C) Schizophrenia is a psychotic disorder, which involves an altered state of reality. Antipsychotic medications are usually effective in treatment of schizophrenia, answer (C). Antianxiety agents are often prescribed for management of symptoms associated with generalized anxiety disorder (GAD) or other varying degrees of anxiety in clients. Hypnotics are prescribed for management of insomnia. Anticonvulsants are used to manage seizure activity caused by various disorders.

Q–319

Eighty-year-old Mr. McKnight returns to the hospital room immediately following orthopedic surgery. Prior to surgery the client was alert and completely oriented. Once back in the room, the client points to an empty windowsill and asks the nurse, "Where did all of those noisy cats come from?" The LPN/LVN understands the client is experiencing

(A) a delusion
(B) a hallucination
(C) paranoia
(D) schizophrenia

Q–320

Following a motor vehicle accident, 17-year-old Simon is paralyzed from the waist down, causing him to be wheelchair bound. Simon later becomes the star on the wheelchair basketball team. This is an example of which of the following?

(A) Denial
(B) Compensation
(C) Displacement
(D) Bargaining

Answers

A–319

(B) A perception by the senses that is unaccounted for by external stimuli is called a hallucination, answer (B). The client is elderly and is still recovering from anesthesia. Hallucinations are not uncommon at this time. A delusion is an inaccurate belief that is not associated with perception of the senses. Paranoia is a disorder that involves persistent delusions of jealousy or personal demise, such as a client constantly thinking that others want to cause him/her harm. Schizophrenia is a disorder involving chronic delusions and hallucinations along with disorganized speech and behavior.

A–320

(B) Simon is making up for his handicap by excelling at an activity. This is an example of compensation, covering up a weakness by overachievement in another area, answer (B). Denial is the refusal to acknowledge a loss or an unacceptable aspect of reality. Displacement involves transferring emotional reactions caused by one object or person onto another. Bargaining is a stage of the grieving process in which the person seeks to avoid loss by offering something in place of whatever is being taken away.

Psychosocial Integrity

Q–321

A student nurse is presenting to the class information on defense mechanisms. The student nurse states, "When a person acts in a way that is exactly opposite to how they feel, it is called _____."

(A) projection
(B) reaction formation
(C) sublimation
(D) substitution

Physiological Integrity:
Pharmacological Therapies

Q–322

Which of the following medications is often prescribed to clients suffering from depression?

(A) Amitriptyline
(B) Alprazolam
(C) Clonazepam
(D) Haloperidol

Answers

A–321

(B) Reaction formation is a defense mechanism that involves actions that are the opposite of what a person actually feels, answer (B). Projection involves blaming other people or objects for whatever is unacceptable. Sublimation is displacing energy associated with primitive drives into acceptable activities or behaviors. Substitution is replacing one object, value, or behavior with another object, value, or behavior that is usually less acceptable, available, or valued.

A–322

(A) Amitriptyline (Elavil) is a medication used to treat depression by increasing effects of serotonin and norepinephrine in the central nervous system (CNS). The correct answer is (A). Alprazolam (Xanax) is an antianxiety agent. Clonazepam (Klonipine) is used to prevent seizure activity caused by various disorders. Haloperidol (Haldol) is an antipsychotic medication.

Physiological Integrity:
Pharmacological Therapies

Q–323

The nurse tells a client recently placed on Dilantin for management of seizure activity that until the physician informs the client otherwise, he must avoid

(A) vigorous exercise
(B) caffeinated beverages
(C) smoking
(D) driving

Health Promotion and Maintenance

Q–324

Mrs. Gregory is a resident with Alzheimer's disease at a nursing facility. Which of the following is a manifestation associated with this disease?

(A) Unsteady gait
(B) Dependence on others for ADLs
(C) Overeating
(D) Loss of childhood memories

A–323

(D) A client who has recently been prescribed Dilantin for control of a seizure disorder should be advised not to drive until the response to the medication is known, answer (D). Prior to driving, the client needs to be seizure free for a period of time determined by the physician. Routine blood tests will be done to ensure therapeutic serum levels of the medication. Clients with seizure disorders should be informed that smoking and caffeine are common triggers of seizure activity, and use of these substances should be monitored.

A–324

(B) Alzheimer's disease is a type of dementia involving a chronic, progressing, and degenerative cognitive impairment. With progression of the disease, clients eventually become dependent on others for assistance in carrying out activities of daily living (ADLs), answer (B). Other symptoms include short-term memory loss, personality changes, and speech difficulties. More severe symptoms, such as seizures and psychosis, can occur in later stages of the disease. Unsteady gait and overeating are not associated with this illness. Memories from the earliest life occurrences are usually retained by the client.

Psychosocial Integrity

Q–325

A client exhibits signs of obsessive-compulsive disorder (OCD). Which of the following best describes the client's pattern of thinking?

(A) Perfectionism
(B) Delusional
(C) Ritualistic
(D) Altered reality

Psychosocial Integrity

Q–326

A 36-year-old male client loses all function from his waist down after sustaining a spinal cord injury after falling off the roof of his house. The nurse asks the client how this injury will affect the different aspects of his life. The client replies, "It won't." This reaction exemplifies that the client is in what stage of the grieving process?

A–325

(C) The client suffering from obsessive-compulsive disorder experiences ritualistic thoughts (OCD). This is a characteristic of the obsessive aspect of OCD. Answer (C) is correct. Perfectionist behaviors are the actions associated with OCD. Delusional thinking and altered reality are manifestations associated with psychotic disorders.

A–326

ANSWER: Denial
RATIONALE: The grieving process involves behavioral responses that represent the following stages: denial, anger, bargaining, depression, and acceptance. Clients usually respond to a loss by following these stages in the order provided. The paralyzed condition of the client is his loss. The client is denying that this loss will affect him or his life.

Physiological Integrity:
Pharmacological Therapies

Q–327

Ativan 0.5 mg IM every 1 hour as needed is prescribed for a client experiencing delirium tremens. The medication vial reads 2mg/mL of solution. How many mL should the LPN/ LVN draw into the syringe for single-dose administration?

Psychosocial Integrity

Q–328

A client going through withdrawal from alcohol is being closely monitored for development of delirium tremens. Which of the following is NOT a symptom of this condition?

(A) Auditory hallucinations
(B) Restlessness
(C) Diaphoresis
(D) Hypotension

Answers

ANSWER: 0.25 mL

RATIONALE: Solve for x mL using the following ratio method.

$$\frac{2 \text{ mg}}{1 \text{ mL}} = \frac{0.5 \text{ mg}}{x \text{ mL}}$$

$$2x = 0.5$$

$$x = \frac{0.5}{2}$$

$$x = 0.25 \text{ mL}$$

(D) Signs of hyperactivity of the autonomic nervous system such as pupillary dilatation, tachycardia, and hypertension are usually present in delirium tremens. The client in this state may experience auditory, visual, and/or tactile hallucinations. Other signs of delirium tremens include extreme disorientation, restlessness, diaphoresis (profuse sweating), and fever.

Psychosocial Integrity

Q–329

A 24-year-old client with anorexia nervosa is admitted to the hospital. Patient care involves close monitoring for which of the following?

(A) Tachycardia
(B) Excessive exercise
(C) Bingeing on food
(D) Elevated serum iron levels

Psychosocial Integrity

Q–330

The LPN/LVN brings daily medications to a paranoid schizophrenic resident at the inpatient psychiatric facility. The client refuses to take the medications stating, "I know you are trying to poison me." Which of the following is an appropriate response by the nurse?

(A) "What makes you think I would be trying to poison you?"
(B) "If you don't take these pills, you may die."
(C) "Your doctor has a good reason for wanting you to take these medications."
(D) "Why would anyone want to poison you?"

Answers

A–329

(B) Patient care for a client with anorexia nervosa involves close and strict monitoring of patient activities. Clients with this disorder often engage themselves in vigorous and excessive exercise, answer (B). Bradycardia is often seen in clients with anorexia nervosa. Bingeing on food is a characteristic of bulimia nervosa. Clients with anorexia nervosa are commonly anemic.

A–330

(A) Using an open-ended question to allow the client to express the reasoning behind the communicated thought is therapeutic and opens the opportunity for intervention. Answer (B) would be threatening to the client and may increase distrust. Answer (C) does not acknowledge the client's fear nor does it promote discussion that could lead to resolution of the underlying issue. Answer (D) does not involve therapeutic use of questioning and may be perceived as insulting to the client.

Psychosocial Integrity

A 23-year-old female client exhibits behaviors of disregard to authority, alcohol and drug abuse, and poor work performance. She has been arrested multiple times for theft and destruction of property. Which of the following are these behaviors characteristic of?

(A) Narcissistic personality disorder
(B) Avoidant personality disorder
(C) Borderline personality disorder
(D) Antisocial personality disorder

Psychosocial Integrity

Suicidal attempts are most commonly made by members of which of the following demographic groups?

(A) Young men
(B) Young women
(C) Older men
(D) Older women

A-331

(D) Antisocial personality disorder involves disregard for the rights of others. Behaviors of this disorder often include acting out against social norms and the law. Narcissistic personality disorder involves behaviors such as fantasizing about unlimited success, power, brilliance, or beauty. Clients with this disorder think that their problems can only be understood by others who are at the same elevated level as themselves. Client behaviors characterized by avoidant personality disorder involve feeling inadequate, oversensitivity to criticism, and social inhibition. Borderline personality disorder includes unpredictable and impulsive behavioral and emotional outbursts.

A-332

(B) Young women are the group that attempt suicide most frequently, answer (B). Suicide is attempted by people of all age groups, whether male or female. Older men who live alone are most likely to be successful at suicide due to the violent methods used for the attempt, such as shooting or hanging themselves. Young women use methods that are fatal at slower rates and more easily correctable, such as ingesting large amounts of medications or cutting their wrists.

Psychosocial Integrity

Q–333

A client admitted to the inpatient psychiatric facility tells a student nurse that she is thinking about committing suicide. Which of the following is the best response by the student?

(A) "Why do you want to kill yourself?"
(B) "Is there something bothering you?"
(C) "Have you determined a way of killing yourself?"
(D) "Maybe you should tell this to your doctor."

Psychosocial Integrity

Q–334

A severely diminished emotional response to a situation, as often seen in clients suffering from depression, is called

(A) poor attitude
(B) blunt affect
(C) flat condition
(D) seasonal affective disorder

A–333

(C) When a client shows signs of suicidal ideation, it is of highest priority to determine the reality of the suicide threat. Clients who have developed a concrete plan for committing suicide are at a higher risk of carrying out the act than those who state they have thought about committing suicide. Answer (C) is the best response. Answer (A) may be threatening to the client. Answer (B) changes the topic, and answer (D) avoids the client's thoughts and feelings and closes the opportunity for intervention. This statement by the client suggests that the client may be in immediate danger. All of the incorrect answers fail to recognize this danger.

A–334

(B) A person with a depressive disorder may be described as having a blunt affect if she or he shows a decreased emotional response to the surrounding condition or situation. A poor attitude is not used to describe behavior or responses of clients. A flat affect, not condition, refers to an absence of emotional response to a situation. Seasonal affective disorder is a condition of low serotonin levels, which normally occur in the winter months or at times when the amount of daily sunlight is low.

Physiological Integrity:
Pharmacological Therapies

Q–335

Which of the following is NOT a classification of medications used to treat affective disorders?

(A) Monoamine oxidase (MAO) inhibitors
(B) Selective serotonin reuptake inhibitors (SSRIs)
(C) Tricyclics
(D) Tetracyclines

Safe and Effective Care Environment:
Coordinated Care

Q–336

In accordance with the "Patient's Bill of Rights," select all of the following that relate to the rights of hospitalized clients.

(A) Confidentiality of all matters pertaining to care
(B) Immediate family members may review medical records
(C) Clients are informed about advanced directives
(D) Any reasonable requested care or services must be provided
(E) All rights must be explained to clients
(F) Continuity of care

Answers

(D) Tetracyclines are a classification of antibiotic. These are not used to treat affective disorders. Affective disorders are also known as depressive disorders. Monoamine oxidase (MAO) inhibitors, selective serotonin reuptake inhibitors (SSRIs), and tricyclics are all classifications of antidepressant agents.

(A), **(C)**, **(D)**, **(E)**, and **(F)** are all correct. Except for answer **(B)**, all of the above pertain to client rights during hospitalization, according to the "Patient's Bill of Rights" published by the American Hospital Association (AHA). This documents rights regarding privacy, considerate and respectful care, autonomous decision making, and advanced directives. The right to privacy includes confidentiality. This means that only the client can request to review his/her own medical records. However, the client may allow medical information to be released to others.

Health Promotion and Maintenance

Q–337

While assessing a 75-year-old client, the nurse is aware that normal changes that occur with age include: (select all that apply)

(A) Skin turgor increases
(B) Subcutaneous fat increases
(C) Decrease in muscle fibers
(D) Blood calcium decreases
(E) Acuity to high-frequency sound increases
(F) Increased pain threshold

Physiological Integrity:
Basic Care and Comfort

Q–338

A client is hospitalized with advanced rheumatic disease. The LPN/LVN knows that prevention of hip flexion contractures includes placing the client in which of the following positions?

(A) Supine
(B) Prone
(C) Side-lying
(D) Fowler's

Answers

(C) and (F) are correct. Many physical changes occur with age. Integumentary changes include increased skin dryness, which decreases skin turgor. Subcutaneous fat decreases, which leads to wrinkling. The number of muscle tissue fibers decreases causing decreased speed and power of skeletal muscle. Calcium is lost from the bones with age, which leads to osteoporosis. Auditory acuity decreases beginning with high-frequency sounds, which leads to progressive hearing loss. Due to changes in neurons and nerve conduction, threshold to pain, touch, and temperature increase with age.

(B) Flexor muscles have more strength than extender muscles. When use of muscles is limited, this leads to the potential development of contractures. Contractures are deformities caused by shortening and fibrosis of connective tissue. To prevent contractures, muscles should be maintained in an extended position. The best position to extend hip muscles is the prone position, answer (B). Supine position is also recommended for clients with rheumatic diseases to prevent kyphosis of the vertebrae. Prolonged lying in side-lying or Fowler's positions promotes flexion contractures.

Physiological Integrity:
Physiological Adaptation

Q–339

Mrs. Spivey is a 60-year-old client with rheumatoid arthritis (RA). The LPN/LVN understands the pathophysiologic process of this disorder to include all of the following factors, except:

(A) RA is an autoimmune disease.
(B) RA causes loss of muscle elasticity and contractility.
(C) RA involves destruction of cartilage and bone.
(D) RA symptoms occur as a result of mechanical injury.

Physiological Integrity:
Pharmacological Therapies

Q–340

Along with non-pharmacologic pain relief measures, initial treatment of osteoarthritis (OA) involves prescribing high doses of which of the following medications?

(A) Aspirin
(B) Acetaminophen
(C) Ibuprofen
(D) Naproxen

A–339

(D) Rheumatoid arthritis (RA) is an autoimmune reaction that occurs in synovial tissue. Enzymes break down tissue in the joint, which ultimately leads to destruction of cartilage and bone tissue. Degeneration of muscle fibers causes loss of muscle elasticity and contractility. All of this results in loss of joint function. Answer (D) is the correct choice. Mechanical injury to joints is the primary factor in development of degenerative joint disease, or osteoarthritis.

A–340

(B) Studies have shown that use of non-steroidal anti-inflammatory drugs (NSAIDs) to treat pain and inflammation associated with osteoarthritis (OA) may increase progression of the breakdown of cartilage. Aspirin, ibuprofen, and naproxen are all NSAIDs that can normally be bought over-the-counter. Answer (B) is correct. Tylenol has shown to be as effective as NSAIDs to treat symptoms of OA and does not cause the degenerative effects that have been identified with NSAID use.

Physiological Integrity:
Pharmacological Therapies

Q–341

Demerol 50 mg IM every 3 hours is prescribed for a post-operative client. This medication is available in a concentration of 75mg/mL. For administration, the LPN/LVN would draw up how much medication in milliliters (mL)?

(A) 1 mL
(B) 0.85 mL
(C) 0.7 mL
(D) 1.5 mL

Health Promotion and Maintenance

Q–342

At birth, a newborn expands the lungs with the first breath, causing changes to the circulation of blood. Fetal circulation differs from postnatal circulation in all of the following ways except:

(A) In a fetus, blood travels from the umbilical vein to the aorta through the ductus venosus.
(B) The ductus arteriosus, which allows passage of blood from the pulmonary artery to the aorta during gestation, closes after birth.
(C) The fetal heart contains an opening between the right and left atria called the foramen ovale.
(D) The umbilical cord transports blood and nutrients between the fetus to the placenta and is composed of one vein and two arteries.

Answers

(C) Solve for x mL using the following ratio method.

$$\frac{75 \text{ mg}}{1 \text{ mL}} = \frac{50 \text{ mg}}{x \text{ mL}}$$

$$75x = 50$$

$$x = \frac{50}{75}$$

$$x = 0.67 \text{ rounded up to } 0.7 \text{ mL}$$

The correct answer is (C).

(A) The ductus venosus is a passageway that allows oxygenated blood from the umbilical vein to enter the inferior vena cava. Blood passes from the pulmonary artery to the descending aorta by way of the ductus arteriosus in fetal circulation. The foramen ovale is an opening between the right atrium and the left atrium of the heart in a fetus. The umbilical cord is cut at birth once respirations have occurred that initiate changes in the circulation of the newborn. The umbilical cord functions in utero as the transport system between the mother and the fetus by way of the placenta. The cord is composed of one vein and two arteries.

Health Promotion and Maintenance

Q–343

Mrs. Perez is visiting the clinic for a prenatal assessment. This is the client's fourth pregnancy. She lost one pregnancy during the ninth week of gestation. One pregnancy resulted in the birth of a stillborn infant at full term, and she has one living child who was born during the 35th week of gestation. Which of the following best describes this client?

(A) Para 4 gravida 1111
(B) Gravida 4 para 1111
(C) Gravida 1 para 4111
(D) Para 1 gravida 4111

Health Promotion and Maintenance

Q–344

RhoGAM (Rh immune globulin) would most likely be administered to which of the following clients after delivery?

(A) An AB+ blood type client within 72 hours after delivery of her newborn
(B) A B+ blood type client with an O– blood type husband
(C) An O– blood type client with titers that show sensitivity to Rh factor
(D) An A– blood type client within 72 hours after spontaneous abortion

Answers

(B) Gravida represents the total number of pregnancies that the client has had. Para describes the results of the pregnancies. Para is made up of four parts: the number of infants born at term or after 37 weeks; the number of infants born preterm or after 20 weeks but before 37 weeks; the number of spontaneous or therapeutic abortions or pregnancies that ended prior to 20 weeks; and the number of living children. Mrs. Perez has had four pregnancies, meaning she is a gravida 4. She gave birth to a stillborn infant at term, gave birth to a preterm infant who is also her living child, and lost one pregnancy during the ninth week of gestation. Mrs. Perez is Gravida 4 Para 1111, answer (B).

(D) RhoGAM (Rh immune globulin) is used to prevent sensitivity to Rh factor in a woman who is Rh negative. Birth of an Rh positive child will cause production of antibodies against Rh factor, which would harm future pregnancies of Rh positive fetuses. Answer (D) is correct. A client with an Rh positive blood type does not need this intervention. The Rh negative father of the fetus does not pose this risk to this or any future pregnancies. Once sensitivity is already present due to production of antibodies against Rh factor, RhoGAM cannot be used and other preventative measures must be taken during pregnancy and birth.

Health Promotion and Maintenance

Q–345

Mrs. Case receives teaching from the LPN/LVN prior to discharge from the hospital regarding normal discharge after vaginal birth. The nurse would have informed the client that from about the third postpartum day until approximately the tenth day, vaginal discharge may

(A) be pink to brownish in color.
(B) be creamy or yellowish.
(C) be dark red in color.
(D) contain large clots.

Health Promotion and Maintenance

Q–346

After emergency Cesarean section delivery, Mrs. Peters has a 7 lb 4 oz newborn baby girl. Once breastfeeding is initiated, the client complains of abdominal cramping. Which of the following is the most appropriate response by the nurse?

(A) "Many new mothers find that breastfeeding is too difficult and switch to bottle feeding."
(B) "Breastfeeding stimulates release of oxytocin, which is a hormone that causes the uterus to contract."
(C) "You are experiencing 'after pains.' I can get you some pain medication, and you can wait until later to breastfeed."
(D) "You may want to try breastfeeding using the 'football hold' to avoid laying the infant directly on the abdominal incision."

Answers

A–345

(A) Lochia serosa, which is pink to brownish in color, is the vaginal discharge noted between three and ten days after vaginal birth. Lochia alba is creamy or yellowish. This discharge begins around postpartum day ten, and continues for about one to two weeks. Lochia rubra is the initial vaginal discharge, which occurs during the first two to three postpartum days. Lochia rubra may contain small clots, but if clots larger than nickel-size are noticed, the physician should be notified.

A–346

(B) Oxytocin is a hormone that promotes release of milk by the mammary glands. This hormone is released after birth to promote uterine contractions, which helps return the uterus back to its normal size. Answer (B) is the best response. The new mother should not be discouraged from breastfeeding, which promotes bonding and is the most complete nutrition available to a newborn. The success rate of breastfeeding increases the earlier this process begins and the more time a mother and newborn have to breastfeed. Pain medication should be provided 30 to 45 minutes prior to initiating breastfeeding. The cramping is most likely caused by uterine contractions, not incisional pain.

Physiological Integrity:
Basic Care and Comfort

Q–347

A client is not allowed anything by mouth (NPO) while testing is being performed to rule out a cerebrovascular accident. The client is placed on an intravenous isotonic solution to maintain hydration. Which of the following is an isotonic solution?

(A) 3% sodium chloride
(B) 0.45% sodium chloride
(C) 5% dextrose in water
(D) 5% dextrose in normal saline

Health Promotion and Maintenance

Q–348

Newborn babies are given an injection on the day of birth to increase blood coagulation factors, which are present in deficient amounts in the neonates' bodies. Which of the following medications does this injection consist of?

(A) Vitamin K
(B) Ferrous sulfate
(C) Erythromycin
(D) RhoGAM

Answers

(C) Isotonic solutions are fluids that are of similar composition to the extracellular fluid of the blood. These solutions are used to increase the amount of circulating blood fluid. Examples of isotonic solutions are 5% dextrose in water (D_5W), Lactated Ringer's, and 0.9% sodium chloride (normal saline). Answer (C) is correct. Three percentage sodium chloride and 5% dextrose in normal saline (D_5NS) are hypertonic solutions. 0.45% sodium chloride is a hypotonic solution.

(A) While in the uterus, the liver is primarily responsible for blood coagulation. After birth, Vitamin K activates the factors produced by the liver that are responsible for blood coagulation. The immature intestinal tract of a newborn does not contain the flora that produces the body's Vitamin K. Therefore, infants are injected with Vitamin K at birth to prevent potential bleeding problems caused by its deficiency. Answer (A) is correct. Ferrous sulfate is used to supplement iron to the body. It is not given to newborns at birth. Erythromycin is an antibiotic ointment applied to the eyes of newborns to prevent eye infections. Rho-GAM is used to prevent Rh sensitization in Rh negative mothers.

Health Promotion and Maintenance

Q–349

Mrs. Anderson has given birth to a full-term baby girl. At birth the infant weighs 6 lbs 3 oz and is 21 inches long. The mother and baby are discharged on the second postpartum day. Mrs. Anderson plans to breastfeed for at least 6 months. The baby girl will be considered a neonate

(A) from birth until 1 year of age
(B) until she is over 7 lbs
(C) until she is no longer breastfed
(D) from birth until she is 28 days old

Psychosocial Integrity

Q–350

A client has been admitted for treatment of a fractured femur that was sustained during an automobile accident caused by the client's alcohol intoxication. The client tells the nurse, "I only had a few drinks to calm myself after a hard day." The nurse knows that this client is using what type of ego defense mechanism to deal with this situation?

(A) Compensation
(B) Denial
(C) Rationalization
(D) Reaction formation

Answers

(D) The neonatal period begins at the time of birth and continues until the 28th day of life, answer (D). From birth until one year of age, the newborn is considered an infant. Neonate represents the age of the newborn. The neonatal period is not determined by weight. The method of feeding the newborn does not determine the neonatal status.

(C) The client is attempting to make excuses or formulate logical reasons to justify unacceptable behaviors, which is the definition of rationalization. Compensation is covering up a real or perceived weakness by emphasizing a trait that is more desirable. Denial is refusing to acknowledge the existence of a real situation or the feelings associated with it. Reaction formation is the prevention of unacceptable thoughts or behaviors from being expressed by exaggerating opposite thoughts or types of behaviors.

Safe and Effective Care Environment:
Coordinated Care

Q–351

A nurse is aware that state boards of nursing hold what primary responsibility?

(A) Approving nursing education programs in the state
(B) Transferring licenses of nurses who are licensed in another state
(C) Protecting the public's health and well-being
(D) Overseeing procedures for licensure exams

Safe and Effective Care Environment:
Coordinated Care

Q–352

A nurse has just finished making rounds with a healthcare provider and says to another nurse, "I don't know why anyone would want him for a healthcare provider, he's a fool." The nurse is at risk for what charge related to this conversation?

(A) Assault
(B) Slander
(C) Libel
(D) Negligence

A–351

(C) State boards of nursing have multiple responsibilities that include review and approval of nursing education programs, issuing and transferring nursing licenses, and overseeing procedures for licensure exams, but the primary responsibility of a state board of nursing is to protect the public's health and well-being.

A–352

(B) A comment uttered aloud that could be construed as a character attack is known as slander. A written comment attacking a person's character is libel. Assault is a threat to do bodily harm to an individual and negligence describes the failure to act as a reasonable person would act in a similar situation.

Safe and Effective Care Environment:
Coordinated Care

Q–353

The nurse is caring for a client who is in wrist restraints that were ordered by the healthcare provider to prevent the client from pulling out the intravenous lines. What is the nurse's most important nursing intervention when caring for this client?

(A) Remove the restraints every 4 hours and perform range of motion exercises to the arms.
(B) Request an order for a sedative medication from the healthcare provider so that the restraints can be removed.
(C) Ensure that the client is taken to the bathroom every 4–6 hours.
(D) Assess the client's well-being every 15–30 minutes.

Safe and Effective Care Environment:
Coordinated Care

Q–354

The nurse is aware that the number of malpractice suits that involve nurses has increased because of which of the following reasons? Select all that apply.

(A) Increased use of licensed nurses at the bedside
(B) Increased use of technology in client care
(C) Clients lack of understanding of malpractice law
(D) Downsizing of healthcare facilities
(E) Early discharge home from healthcare facilities

Answers

A–353

(D) A client who is in restraints is not able to protect himself or provide for his own needs. The most important nursing intervention is to assess the client frequently and provide what is needed after these assessments. Restraints should be removed every 2 hours and the nurse should offer to take the client to the bathroom more frequently than every 4–6 hours. Asking for an order for a sedative is not appropriate because this would not prevent the client from pulling at the IV lines and it may compromise the client's respiratory effort.

A–354

(B), **(D)**, and **(E)** Several factors have contributed to the increased number of malpractice suits against nurses. These factors include: delegation of more tasks to UAPs, early discharge of clients, shortage of professional nurses and past downsizing of hospitals, technological advances that require greater expertise, better informed consumers, and an expanded definition of liability.

Psychosocial Integrity

Q–355

The nurse is caring for an 88-year old male client who was admitted with a urinary tract infection. The client, who lives with his nephew, is mobile and provides most of his own care but recently developed confusion and incontinence. The nephew told the nurse that he couldn't continue to take care of the client if he remains incontinent. What aspects of this client's history are risk factors for elder abuse? Select all that apply.

(A) Client is 88.
(B) Client is male.
(C) Client is mobile.
(D) Client lives with his nephew.
(E) Client has developed confusion and incontinence.

Physiological Integrity

Q–356

The nurse is caring for four geriatric clients and will observe which client most closely for suicidal ideation?

(A) A 72-year-old female who babysits her grandchildren three times per week
(B) An 84-year-old male who has coffee every morning with a group of retirees
(C) A 79-year-old male whose wife of 60 years died two months ago and has no children
(D) A 90-year-old female who drives to church every morning for a worship service

A–355

(**A**) and (**E**) Identified risk factors for victims of abuse included being a white female age 70 or older, being mentally or physically impaired, being unable to meet daily self-care needs, and having care needs that exceeded the caretaker's ability.

A–356

(**C**) It is felt that increasing social isolation is a contributing factor to suicide among the elderly. Men seem especially vulnerable after the loss of a spouse. The other clients are not affected by social isolation.

Psychosocial Integrity

Q–357

The nurse is caring for a client who is admitted with major depression. Which statements by the nurse are the best assessments for suicidal ideation? Select all that apply.

(A) "Would you like to talk to me about why you are feeling so sad?"
(B) "Do you have any plans for hurting yourself?"
(C) "Wouldn't you like to try to feel better?"
(D) "What do you think made you feel so sad this time?"
(E) "Have you ever had a time in your life when you attempted suicide?"

Physiological Integrity

Q–358

The nurse is caring for a seven-year-old client with autism spectrum disorder who has been admitted to the pediatric unit after an emergency appendectomy. What nursing interventions would best address the client's needs presented by the autism spectrum disorder diagnosis? Select all that apply.

(A) Limit the number of individuals who provide care for the child.
(B) Restrict the child's access to familiar objects.
(C) Keep the television in the room on at all times.
(D) Address all instructions and questions to the parents.
(E) Follow the child's usual schedule as much as possible.

Answers

A–357

(**B**) and (**E**) The nurse must ask direct questions if there is suspicion of suicidal ideation. The nurse should assess if the client has ever thought of harming himself, ever acted on a plan, or ever attempted suicide before. The other statements would not provide information about the client's thoughts or plans of suicide.

A–358

(**A**) and (**E**) Even minor changes in the environment of an individual with autism spectrum disorder may be met with resistance or hysterical responses. The client should have a limited number of caregivers assigned to provide care. The nurse should provide whatever familiar objects the child needs to feel safe. The nurse should work to limit excess stimulation so the TV should not be left on constantly unless that is normal for the child. Even if the child is nonverbal, it is important for the nurse to address the child and provide instructions and give the child the opportunity to answer questions. It is also very helpful if the routines of the healthcare facility are as close as possible to the home environment.

Q–359

A nurse is working in a child care center and notices that one child has had a broken arm and a black eye in the past six months. This child also has consistent bruises that are consistent with the child being held tightly. What is the nurse's best action if it is believed that this child is being abused?

(A) The nurse does not have to report anything because there is no proof the child is being abused.
(B) The nurse should report the suspicion to the administrator of the child care center.
(C) The nurse should call the state child welfare agency and report the suspicion.
(D) The nurse should question the child to determine if the child reports abuse.

Q–360

The LPN/LVN is caring for a client in an emergency care clinic who is complaining of a severe headache. The healthcare provider tells the nurse to give the client 1.5 mL of sterile saline as an IM injection because this client is seen frequently with this same complaint. What are the LPN/LVN's best options in this situation? Select all that apply.

(A) Administer the saline because the client is a drug seeker.
(B) Notify the RN who supervises the LPN/LVN.
(C) Send the client to another healthcare facility.
(D) Request that the healthcare provider prescribe an alternative to the saline.
(E) Report the healthcare provider for improper care of the client.

A–359

(C) The nurse has the duty to report any suspicion of abuse. The nurse can't ignore it, and asking the child about any abuse may or may not be productive because the child may attempt to protect the abuser. The nurse would notify the administrator of the child care facility, but the first duty is to report the suspicion to the child welfare agency that handles possible child abuse.

A–360

(B) and (D) While it has been shown that a placebo is effective if the client believes it is effective, the nurse should only administer a placebo if the client agrees to its administration. The LPN/LVN should notify the RN of the healthcare provider's order. It would also be correct for the LPN/LVN to advocate for the client with the healthcare provider by requesting that an alternative medication be prescribed to the client. It is not LPN/LVN's role to suggest that the client go somewhere else for care, and prescribing a placebo, while not considered ethical by some, is not providing improper care.

Safe and Effective Care Environment:
Coordinated Care

Q–361

The nurse is documenting information about a client on a computer in the hall when the nurse is called away to another client. What should the nurse do concerning the documentation that has not been completed?

(A) Log off the computer and complete the documentation at a later time.
(B) Leave the computer logged on, quickly complete the other task, and then return to the computer.
(C) Complete the documentation and then go and see about the other issue.
(D) Complete the documentation and ask an unlicensed assistive personnel (UAP) to check on the other client.

Safe and Effective Care Environment:
Coordinated Care

Q–362

The nurse is caring for a client with dementia who cries and moans all night. The nurse says to the client while holding on to the client's arm, "There is nothing wrong with you. If you don't be quiet I'm going to give you a shot that will keep you from crying ever again." What action has the nurse committed against this client? Choose all that apply.

(A) Assault
(B) Battery
(C) Libel
(D) False imprisonment
(E) Invasion of privacy

Answers

A–361

(A) As important as documentation is, care of clients is more important. Therefore, the nurse should complete the documentation at a later time. It is most important the nurse log off the computer because it is in the hall and unless the nurse logs off, the information on the computer screen could be seen by individuals who are not authorized to view it. The nurse should never leave the computer logged on, even for a few minutes, because it may compromise client confidentiality. The nurse should log off and check on the client, and then if necessary, ask a UAP to assist the client.

A–362

(A) and (B) Assault is an action that places a person in immediate fear of personal violence or offensive contact. It must include words expressing an intention to cause harm and some type of action. Battery occurs when the nurse makes physical contact without a client's consent, which the nurse did by holding on to the client's arm. Libel is a written form of defamation of character. False imprisonment occurs when a client is restrained without legal authorization. The nurse did not violate the client's right to privacy.

Safe and Effective Care Environment:
Safety and Infection Control

Q–363

The nurse is caring for a client who is at risk for the development of severe sepsis and will monitor this client for which manifestations of this life-threatening complication of an infection? Select all that apply.

(A) Hypertension
(B) Oliguria
(C) Lactic acidosis
(D) Hypervigilance
(E) Organ failure

Safe and Effective Care Environment:
Safety and Infection Control

Q–364

The LPN/LVN will reinforce teaching to a client about which ways to prevent tick borne illnesses?

(A) Take a hot shower as soon as he or she comes indoors.
(B) Apply insect repellent before sunscreen.
(C) Wear dark-colored clothing.
(D) Tuck pant legs into socks.

A-363

(B), **(C)**, and **(E)** Severe sepsis is associated with organ dysfunction, hypotension, and hypoperfusion manifested by lactic acidosis, oliguria, and acute alteration in mental status such as confusion and delirium, not hypervigilence.

A-364

(D) There are many things that can be done to prevent tick-borne illnesses. The client should apply sunscreen before insect repellent and wear light-colored clothing because ticks are attracted to dark clothing. The client should undress completely and inspect the body for ticks using mirrors immediately after coming in from the outside. A hot shower will not remove ticks. The client should wear long sleeves and long pants with socks pulled over the pant legs.

Safe and Effective Care Environment:
Safety and Infection Control

Q–365

The nurse is caring for a group of clients. Which medications will increase a client's risk of falling? Select all that apply.

(A) Diazepam
(B) Clonidine
(C) Propranolol
(D) Ciprofloxacin
(E) Methadone

Safe and Effective Care Environment:
Safety and Infection Control

Q–366

The nurse is most at risk for back injury when doing which nursing activities? Select all that apply.

(A) Using a manual client-lift device
(B) Changing linens on the client's bed
(C) Repositioning the client in the chair
(D) Picking up a towel that dropped to the floor
(E) Assisting the client from the toilet to the wheelchair

Answers

(A), (B), (C), and (E) Medications that increase a client's risk of falling include antihypertensives (clonidine and propranolol), sedatives (diazepam), and opioid analgesics (methadone). Most antibiotics (ciprofloxacin) usually don't cause dizziness or light-headedness.

(B), (C), and (E) The activities that cause the most stress to a nurse's back are transferring clients from toilet to chair, weighing clients, lifting clients, lifting a client in bed, repositioning clients in bed or chairs, and changing bed linens. Nurses are encouraged to move clients with a client-lift device (either manual or electric). Nurses incur damage by picking up heavy objects from the floor, not lightweight ones such as towels.

Safe and Effective Care Environment:
Coordinated Care

Q–367

The nurse enters a client's room to obtain a signature for informed consent of a surgical procedure that is to be performed that day. As the nurse places the form in front of the client, the client says, "Today is a perfect day for a drive in the country. I really like peach pie. Have you seen my mother?" What is the nurse's best action in this situation?

(A) Call the next-of-kin listed in the client's chart and ask them to come in and sign the consent.
(B) Immediately inform the client's surgeon about the client's mental status.
(C) Inform the supervisor and request guidance.
(D) Ask the client, "Do you know you are having surgery today?"

Safe and Effective Care Environment:
Coordinated Care

Q–368

The nurse is admitting a client who has a cough with blood-tinged sputum and night sweats. The admitting healthcare provider notes that the client may have tuberculosis. What is the nurse's first action in caring for this client?

(A) Complete the ordered Mantoux skin test on the client.
(B) Obtain the ordered sputum specimen.
(C) Place the client in airborne isolation.
(D) Send the client for the ordered chest x-ray.

A–367

(B) The nurse's duty concerning informed consent is to verify that the client is capable of signing the form and obtain the client's signature on the form. The client in this situation shows a lack of awareness of the hospital environment and should not sign a form for surgery. The nurse should immediately inform the surgeon of the client's mental status and inability to sign. It is the physician's responsibility to explain the procedure to an individual responsible for that client. The nurse does not need to contact the supervisor for further guidance or to see if the client knows that a surgery is scheduled for that day.

A–368

(C) Tuberculosis is a contagious disease and the client should be immediately isolated from other clients and staff until the diagnosis can be confirmed or denied. Once this occurs, the nurse can administer the skin test and obtain the sputum specimen. The chest x-ray can be accomplished in the client's room or the client will be sent to x-ray wearing a special mask.

Safe and Effective Care Environment:
Coordinated Care

Q–369

The nurse in an acute care facility utilizes which methods that are quality-of-care indicators? Select all that apply.

(A) Using a clinical pathway for a common procedure such as a hip replacement
(B) Obtaining a urine specimen on all clients admitted to the healthcare facility
(C) Working with a case manager to organize care among the healthcare disciplines
(D) Initiating common healthcare provider orders if a client develops a complication
(E) Ensuring that all clients have an assessment of vital signs every four hours

Safe and Effective Care Environment:
Coordinated Care

Q–370

The nurse is caring for a client who had a total hip replacement. What member of the healthcare team will assist the client in learning how to put on his own socks and shoes while he is recovering from the surgery?

(A) Physical therapist
(B) Registered nurse
(C) Licensed Practical/Vocational Nurse
(D) Occupational therapist

Answers

A–369

(A), (C), and (D) Methods that have been developed to improve quality of care include clinical pathways for common procedures or diagnoses. Other methods include client satisfaction surveys, quality-of-life questionnaires, functional assessment tools, the use of case management and tracking hospital admissions, morbidity and deaths for clients with chronic illnesses. It has been determined that urine specimens should be reserved for those clients whose condition indicates a need for one and it has also been shown that if possible, clients should be disturbed as little as possible at night.

A–370

(D) An occupational therapist assists a client in relearning tasks that are needed for activities of daily living or for tasks that are needed for work. A physical therapist assists a client in issues such as mobility and gait and muscle strengthening exercises. It is not in either the RN or the LPN/LVN's scope of practice to teach a client how to learn to use adaptive equipment. The nurse may assist in performing these tasks but is not responsible to teach the client how to do it.

Safe and Effective Care Environment:
Safety and Infection Control

Q–371

Which clients are most at risk for falls while hospitalized? Select all that apply.

(A) An 8-day-old infant admitted with possible sepsis
(B) A 17-month-old toddler admitted with respiratory syncytial virus
(C) A 15-year-old teen admitted for an emergency appendectomy
(D) A 45-year-old adult admitted with community acquired pneumonia
(E) A 79-year-old adult admitted with dehydration caused by diarrhea

Safe and Effective Care Environment:
Safety and Infection Control

Q–372

The nurse is caring for the following clients. Which clients are most at risk for injury? Select all that apply.

(A) A 22-year-old client admitted after a cholecystectomy who is blind
(B) A 37-year-old client admitted with a fractured femur who has a prior history of depression
(C) A 59-year-old client admitted with a dysrhythmia who speaks English as a second language
(D) A 62-year-old client admitted after a thyroidectomy who stopped smoking 3 months ago
(E) A 74-year-old client admitted after a stroke who has early signs of dementia

Answers

(**B**) and (**E**) While all clients are at risk for falls in the hospital due to the unfamiliar environment and IV lines, pumps, and oxygen tubing, some clients are more at risk than others. A toddler is at high risk because of his developmental ability. The toddler is able to walk and climb but does not have a fear of falling. The older adult has slower reflexes, decreased muscle strength and joint mobility, and the need to use the bathroom quickly (due to diarrhea), all of which predispose this client to falls. An 8-day-old infant has a risk of falling, but at this age has limited ability to turn and roll. A teenager and a 45-year-old adult have the least risk of falling.

(**A**), (**B**), and (**E**) Clients who are most at risk for injury are those who have problems with cognition, sensory and perceptual problems, impaired communication, impaired mobility, loss of physical and emotional well-being, and a lack of safety awareness. The client who is blind, the client who has a fractured femur, and the client who has dementia are most at risk for injury.

Safe and Effective Care Environment:
Safety and Infection Control

Q–373

A school nurse is leading a group discussion concerning safety with a group of high school students. Which topics are most important for the nurse to focus on? Select all that apply.

(A) Wearing seat belts in a motor vehicle
(B) Workplace injuries
(C) Dangers of alcohol and drugs
(D) Reducing sport-related injuries
(E) Fall risk

Safe and Effective Care Environment:
Safety and Infection Control

Q–374

The nurse is caring for a client who has a history of violence toward healthcare workers. What is the nurse's best action to prevent this client from becoming violent again?

(A) Medicate the client with an antipsychotic drug.
(B) Attempt to discover what is causing the client anxiety.
(C) Obtain an order from the healthcare provider to place the client in wrist restraints.
(D) Always make sure that at least three healthcare workers are in the client's room when care is given.

A–373

(A), **(C)**, and **(D)** The leading cause of death in the adolescent and teenager is motor vehicle accidents, followed by homicides, which are both influenced by alcohol and drug use. People in this age group also experience sports and recreational injuries. They commonly feel indestructible, which makes them prone to injury through risk-taking behavior. Workplace injuries are common in the adult population and an increased incidence of falls occurs in the older adult.

A–374

(B) Violence typically begins with anxiety and escalates in stages through verbal aggression and then to physical aggression. If the nurse can relieve the client's anxiety, this may be able to halt the progression to physical violence. Medicating the client or restraining the client's wrists will not decrease the client's tendency to violence, and it is not feasible to have three people in the client's room every time care is needed.

Safe and Effective Care Environment:
Safety and Infection Control

Q–375

The nurse is concerned that a client may become violent. What factors in the client's history or physical condition may increase the risk for aggression? Select all that apply.

(A) The client has schizophrenia.
(B) The client's vital signs are T-98.9° F., BP 150/90, R-18, P-102.
(C) The client's last alcoholic drink was 10 hours ago.
(D) The client was admitted with a possible skull fracture.
(E) The client has a history of syncope.

Safe and Effective Care Environment:
Coordinated Care

Q–376

The nurse is caring for four clients who are receiving chemotherapy for cancer. After reviewing the laboratory results of these clients, which client would the nurse assess first?

(A) The client with a Hgb of 8.9 g/dL
(B) The client with a WBC of 3,900 mm³
(C) The client with a platelet count of 3,000/mm³
(D) The client with a Hct of 32%

A–375

(A), (C), and (D) The factors that increase the risk for aggression include mental disorders such as dementia, delirium, schizophrenia. and bipolar disorder; being under the influence of alcohol or other drugs or being in withdrawal from alcohol or other drugs; and a history of violence and clinical conditions such as high fever, epilepsy head trauma, and hypoglycemia. An elevated blood pressure and a history of syncope would not be risk factors for aggression.

A–376

(C) Though all of the laboratory results are abnormal, a client with a platelet count of 3,000/mm³ is at high risk for a bleeding episode. Normal platelet count is 150,000–450,000/mm³. The Hgb and the Hct are slightly decreased as is the WBC, but the nurse would need to assess the client with the low platelet count first to ensure that the client is not experiencing any acute bleeding episode.

Safe and Effective Care Environment:
Coordinated Care

Q–377

The nurse is caring for four clients with heart disease. Which client will require the most frequent assessment?

(A) An 88-year-old client with right-sided heart failure
(B) An 82-year-old client with tricuspid valve failure
(C) A 76-year-old client with pulmonic valve failure
(D) A 69-year-old client with left-sided heart failure

Safe and Effective Care Environment:
Coordinated Care

Q–378

A nurse is caring for a client who experienced a fall while attempting to get out of bed. In completing the incident report related to the fall, the nurse knows that this information will be used for what primary purpose?

(A) To determine if the nurse could have prevented the fall
(B) To document the personnel involved in the client's care
(C) To gather data to prevent further client falls
(D) To use for future punitive action against the nurse caring for the client

A–377

(**D**) The client with left-sided heart failure will develop pulmonary symptoms much more easily because the blood is unable to leave the left side of the heart and blood backs up into the lungs. The client with right-sided heart failure experiences edema in the periphery of the body, which is not as life threatening as edema of the lungs. The tricuspid valve and the pulmonic valve are located on the right side of the heart and would produce symptoms similar to right-sided heart failure.

A–378

(**C**) The incident report is a tool that is used to document errors or events in the client's stay that may or did cause harm to the client. It is the primary tool of risk management, which seeks to review problems, identify the common elements, and then develop methods to reduce the risk of their occurrence. It is not used to determine fault or used for punitive action. Though it does document the personnel involved in the incident, that is not the primary purpose of the tool.

Psychosocial Integrity

A nurse is called by a neighbor who reports that her teenage son is acting very strangely. The son has nausea and vomiting, has a runny nose, is yawning constantly, and has dilated pupils. The nurse requests the neighbor call for emergency assistance because the son is most likely dealing with what problem?

(A) Opioid intoxication
(B) Opioid withdrawal
(C) Stimulant intoxication
(D) Stimulant withdrawal

Psychosocial Integrity

A nurse works in a sexual abuse center for women. She will make what response to a female client who enters the clinic and reports that she has been raped by her boyfriend?

(A) "How long have you known your boyfriend?"
(B) "I'm so sorry that this happened to you."
(C) "Has this ever happened to you before?"
(D) "I hope you stay away from this man forever."

A–379

(B) Symptoms of opioid withdrawal include nausea, vomiting, diarrhea, rhinorrhea, and dilated pupils. Symptoms of opioid intoxication include euphoria, psychomotor agitation or retardation, and pupillary constriction. Symptoms of stimulant intoxication are tachycardia, pupil dilation, and euphoria. Symptoms of stimulant withdrawal include depression, nightmares, hunger, sweating, and headache.

A–380

(B) It is important for the nurse to communicate some specific concepts to the client who has been raped. These include that the client is safe, that the nurse is sorry that this happened, that the nurse is glad that the client survived, and that this incident is not the client's fault. It is very important that the nurse does not place any blame on the client for the rape.

Psychosocial Integrity

Q–381

The nurse is in the day room of a mental health unit when a client begins to experience symptoms of a panic attack. Which interventions would be most helpful to this client? Select all that apply.

(A) Encourage other clients in the day room to talk to the client.
(B) Speak loudly so that the client is able to hear the instruction of the nurse.
(C) Escort the client to a quiet environment.
(D) Continuously talk to the client until the panic attack is over.
(E) Stay with the client until the panic attack has passed.

Physiological Integrity

Q–382

The nurse is caring for a young woman who suddenly became unable to use her legs. She doesn't appear worried about this sudden onset of paralysis. All diagnostic tests show no physical abnormality. The nurse is aware that the client is most likely dealing with what somatic disorder?

(A) Factitious disorder
(B) Conversion disorder
(C) Illness anxiety disorder
(D) Somatic symptom disorder

Answers

(C) and (E) When a client experiences panic level anxiety, the nurse should stay with the client and offer reassurance and security. Keep the immediate surroundings low in stimuli with dim lighting, few people, and simple décor. Use simple words and brief messages that are spoken calmly and clearly.

(B) The client is exhibiting signs of conversion disorder. In this disorder, the individual suddenly develops a sudden neurological problem such as paralysis, blindness, or the inability to speak. No known physiological reason can be found for the problem. The client displays the classic lack of concern for the problem, "la belle indifference." It is a physiological response to something that causes the client severe anxiety. Factitious disorder involves conscious, intentional pretending to have physical or psychological symptoms. Clients with illness anxiety disorder have an unrealistic or inaccurate interpretation of physical symptoms that leads to preoccupation with a serious disease. Clients with somatic symptom disorder have multiple somatic symptoms that can't be explained medically. Symptoms are vague, dramatized, or exaggerated and the client spends an excessive amount of time and energy devoted to worrying about the symptoms.

Psychosocial Integrity

Q–383

The nurse is caring for a client who is in the manic phase of bipolar disorder. What foods would be most appropriate to place on the client's tray? Select all that apply.

(A) Chicken nuggets
(B) Creamed corn
(C) Carrot sticks
(D) Baked potato
(E) Cupcake

Safe and Effective Care Environment:
Coordinated Care

Q–384

The nurse is caring for four clients with cirrhosis of the liver. Which client will require the most frequent assessments?

(A) The client with a temperature of 100.7° F
(B) The client with ankle edema
(C) The client with purpura
(D) The client with epistaxis

A–383

(A), (C), and (E) Clients who are having a manic episode have a difficult time sitting long enough to eat so the nurse should ensure that the client is provided finger foods that can be easily and safely eaten while the client is walking around. The other foods require the client to sit at a table to consume the food.

A–384

(C) All of the client symptoms require frequent assessments but a mild fever, ankle edema, and epistaxis are all clinical manifestations of compensated cirrhosis. Purpura indicates the client is experiencing a low platelet count and is a manifestation of decompensation, thus requiring the most frequent assessments.

Q–385

The nurse is caring for a client with esophageal varices who begins to experience massive bleeding. What is the most important nursing intervention for the client at this time?

(A) Have the client sign a consent form for an endoscopy.
(B) Prepare to administer blood products.
(C) Encourage the client to swallow frequently.
(D) Ensure that the client has a patent airway.

Q–386

The nurse is assisting the healthcare provider in performing a paracentesis on a client with ascites. What nursing assessments will be most important for the nurse to perform during and immediately after the procedure? Select all that apply.

(A) Oral temperature
(B) Blood pressure
(C) Pulse
(D) Oxygen saturation
(E) Urine output

Answers

(D) Massive bleeding from esophageal varices may cause respiratory compromise because the bleeding may occlude the client's airway. Therefore, before any other procedures are done to treat the client's bleeding episode, the nurse must ensure that the client's airway is patent.

(B) and (E) During and immediately after an abdominal paracentesis, the nurse should monitor blood pressure and urine output to evaluate the effects of fluid shifts that occur during the procedure. Pulse, temperature, and oxygen saturation will be checked before and after the procedure, but the blood pressure and urine output are the most important assessments for this client.

Safe and Effective Care Environment:
Coordinated Care

Q–387

The nurse is caring for a client with Cushing's disease. Which nursing action is most important in the care of this client?

(A) Frequent hand hygiene
(B) Blood pressure assessment
(C) Decreased environmental stimuli
(D) Monitor fluid intake

Safe and Effective Care Environment:
Coordinated Care

Q–388

The LPN/LVN has been assigned to assist with individuals who are being brought to the emergency department of the healthcare facility after a serious bus accident. The LPN/LVN will most likely assist with the care of accident victims with what color triage tag?

(A) Red
(B) Yellow
(C) Green
(D) Black

Answers

A–387

(A) A client with Cushing's disease is at high risk of infection because of the immunosuppression caused by the adrenal tumor. It is therefore most important to perform frequent hand hygiene to protect the client from infection. This action is more important than assessing the blood pressure, decreasing the environmental stimuli, and monitoring fluid intake.

A–388

(B) The LPN/LVN will most likely be assigned to care for accident victims with yellow tags. Yellow indicates the victim has a serious injury but is stable and treatment may be delayed up to six to eight hours. Victims with red tags have life-threatening but survivable injuries as long as treatment is given rapidly. Victims with red tags will most likely be assigned to RNs. Victims with a green tag have minor injuries that can wait longer than eight hours for treatment and will likely be cared for by unlicensed assistive personnel or volunteers. Victims with a black tag are expected to die soon and because of limited resources are not given care.

Safe and Effective Care Environment:
Coordinated Care

Q–389

The nurse is caring for four clients with a metabolic disorder. After reviewing blood gas results, which client will the nurse see first?

(A) pH of 7.33, HCO_3 of 20 mEq/L, and $PaCO_2$ of 43 mm Hg
(B) pH of 7.36, HCO_3 of 21 mEq/L, and $PaCO_2$ of 33 mm Hg
(C) pH of 7.46, HCO_3 of 27 mEq/L, and $PaCO_2$ of 48 mm Hg
(D) pH of 7. 43, HCO_3 of 23 mEq/L, and $PaCO_2$ of 47 mm Hg

Safe and Effective Care Environment:
Safety and Infection Control

Q–390

The nurse knows that it is best to use soap and water for hand hygiene instead of hand sanitizer in which situation?

(A) Before putting on gloves
(B) After administering an oral medication
(C) Before feeding a client
(D) After obtaining a urine specimen

Answers

A–389

(A) The client who needs to be seen first is the client who has uncompensated metabolic acidosis. That client would have a pH less than 7.35, an HCO_3 < 22 mEq/L, and a normal (35–45 mm Hg) $PaCO_2$. The other blood gas results indicate either a partially compensated or a compensated form of metabolic acidosis or metabolic alkalosis.

A–390

(D) Soap and water is used when there is visible soil in the hands and when in contact with body fluids. Hand sanitizer is used at all other times.

Safe and Effective Care Environment:
Safety and Infection Control

Q–391

The LPN/LVN has assigned personal care to an unlicensed assistive personnel (UAP) of a client in contact isolation. What action by the UAP would cause the LPN/LVN to immediately counsel the UAP?

(A) The UAP removes the contaminated gloves first.
(B) The UAP leaves the client's room wearing contaminated gloves, gown, and face shield.
(C) The UAP disposes of the client's soiled linens in a hamper stored in the client's room.
(D) The UAP performs hand hygiene as soon as all personal protective equipment is removed.

Safe and Effective Care Environment:
Safety and Infection Control

Q–392

The LPN/LVN is caring for a 94-year-old client who was admitted with a urinary tract infection and will notify the RN about the possible development of sepsis in this client if the client manifests which symptoms? Select all that apply.

(A) Temperature between 98.7 and 100.3° F.
(B) Heart rate greater than 90 beats/minute.
(C) WBCs greater than 12,000 cells/mm³
(D) Respiratory rate less than 10 breaths/min.
(E) Peripheral oxygen saturation between 95 and 98%

Answers

A-391

(B) The nurse would intervene immediately if the UAP left the client's room wearing contaminated PPE because it could spread infection from the client to other clients on the unit. The UAP is correct to remove gloves first, dispose of soiled linens in the proper container in the client's room, and perform hand hygiene as soon as all PPE is removed.

A-392

(B) and (C) The client with an existing infection may be developing sepsis if the client has two or more of the following characteristics: Temp greater than 100.4° F or less than 96.8° F, a heart rate greater than 90 beats/minute, WBCs greater than 12,000 mm Hg, and a respiratory rate greater than 20 breaths/min or a $PaCO_2$ less than 32 mm Hg.

Safe and Effective Care Environment:
Coordinated Care

Q–393

A nurse cared for a client who refused all efforts to provide personal care while hospitalized. Approximately one year after the client was discharged from the hospital, the client filed suit against the hospital and the staff that cared for him, claiming that he was neglected during his hospitalization. What client actions will be most useful to the nurse during this lawsuit?

(A) Client refused morning care.
(B) Client states, "I don't want anyone touching me. Go away. I'll get my own bath."
(C) Client does not want a bath or linen changed this morning.
(D) Client appears unhappy to be in the hospital and states, "I want to go home."

Safe and Effective Care Environment:
Coordinated Care

Q–394

Which ethical value is the nurse demonstrating when he or she calls the healthcare provider and states, "Mr. H has an order to be discharged today but he has not fully mastered glucose self-monitoring or self-injection of insulin."

(A) Fidelity
(B) Justice
(C) Nonmaleficence
(D) Beneficence

A–393

(B) The best defense against lawsuits is to be very complete in documentation. The nurse should, as much as possible, use the client's own words to describe any issues that are encountered, especially if the client refuses care. The court will read the nurse's documentation that shows that the client refused to be touched and said he would take care of bathing himself.

A–394

(D) Beneficence is the duty to do good for the clients assigned to the nurse's care. It directly supports the nurse's role of client advocate, which is safeguarding a client's rights and supporting their interests. Fidelity is the duty to maintain commitments of professional obligations and responsibilities. Justice is the duty to be fair to all people and nonmaleficence is the duty to do no harm to the client.

Safe and Effective Care Environment:
Coordinated Care

Q–395

The nurse uses ethical principles in caring for all clients. Which client situation illustrates the nurse demonstrating nonmaleficence?

(A) The nurse promises the client to return in 20 minutes to check on the client.

(B) The nurse administers an antibiotic to cure a client's infection that also makes the client nauseated.

(C) The nurse supports the client's decision to stop all treatment for kidney failure.

(D) The nurse tells the client his blood pressure even when it is elevated.

Safe and Effective Care Environment:
Coordinated Care

Q–396

The nurse is caring for the following four clients. Which client will require the most frequent assessments?

(A) The client recently diagnosed with Guillain-Barré syndrome

(B) The client with type 1 diabetes mellitus who will be discharged tomorrow

(C) The client with gastroenteritis who is receiving intravenous rehydration therapy

(D) The client with rheumatoid arthritis who has an acute inflammation of the knee

Answers

(B) Nonmaleficence is the duty to do no harm to the client and involves administering a treatment that is ethically correct (medication to cure an infection) even though the medication causes the client to feel ill. Returning at the promised time demonstrates fidelity, supporting the client's decision to stop treatment is autonomy, and telling the client the results of a test (blood pressure measurement) is veracity.

(A) Guillain-Barré syndrome is an autoimmune disorder that causes ascending paralysis. The disease can progress in a matter of hours from tingling and numbness in the feet to paralysis of the client's diaphragm, so it is important to frequently assess the client's condition. A client who is being discharged tomorrow, a client with gastroenteritis, and a client with rheumatoid arthritis would not need as frequent assessments as the client with Guillain-Barré.

Safe and Effective Care Environment:
Coordinated Care

Q–397

The nurse is caring for four clients who have an opportunistic infection related to AIDS. Which of these clients will require the most frequent assessments?

(A) The client with cryptosporidiosis
(B) The client with AIDS dementia complex
(C) The client with *Pneumocystis carinii* pneumonia
(D) The client with candidiasis

Safe and Effective Care Environment:
Safety and Infection Control

Q–398

The nurse is caring for a client who has developed Vancomycin-resistant enterococci (VRE) infection. Which risk factors are associated with the development of this antibiotic resistance? Select all that apply.

(A) Client had a urinary catheter for the last 48 hours.
(B) Client had a central intravenous catheter placed six days ago.
(C) Client has taken prednisone for the last two years.
(D) Client had a broken arm two years ago.
(E) Client is an insulin-dependent diabetic.

A–397

(C) Pneumocystis pneumonia can become so severe that it causes respiratory failure and mechanical ventilation, which will require the nurse to monitor the client frequently for worsening respiratory changes. Cryptosporidiosis causes diarrhea and fluid loss, and the client with AIDS dementia complex will both require frequent assessment but not as frequent as the client with pneumocystis. The client with candidiasis needs regular assessments.

A–398

(B) and **(C)** Clients who are at increased risk of becoming infected with VRE are clients who have previously had long-term antibiotic treatment, are hospitalized, have a weakened immune system, have undergone surgical procedures, and have long-term devices such as urinary catheters and central intravenous catheters.

Safe and Effective Care Environment:
Safety and Infection Control

Q–399

The nurse knows that a client who takes which medication is most at risk for developing an infection?

(A) Phenytoin
(B) Prednisone
(C) Metoprolol
(D) Alprazolam

Safe and Effective Care Environment:
Safety and Infection Control

Q–400

The nurse is caring for a female client who has developed a vaginal yeast infection as a result of treatment with which other medication?

(A) Reserpine
(B) Amoxicillin
(C) Buspirone
(D) Nadolol

Answers

A–399

(B) Prednisone is a medication used for many things including decreased inflammatory response and immunosuppression. When a client takes this medication, the risk of infection is greatly increased. Phenytoin, metoprolol, and alprazolam do not cause immunosuppression.

A–400

(B) Antibiotics can cause a vaginal yeast infection because the drug destroys colonies of normal vaginal flora, allowing the harmful microbes to thrive. Reserpine, buspirone, and nadolol will not cause a superinfection.

Safe and Effective Care Environment:
Safety and Infection Control

Q–401

The nurse is aware that an elevated temperature may not occur in the presence of infection in which clients? Select all that apply.

(A) A client who is receiving chemotherapy
(B) A client with diabetes
(C) A client who is 88 years old
(D) A client with heart failure
(E) A client with malnutrition

Safe and Effective Care Environment:
Coordinated Care

Q–402

A nurse has been subpoenaed to give a deposition in a case a former client filed against the hospital and all of the staff that cared for him while in the hospital. What is the nurse's best response to the following question by the lawyer, "Did you provide care to Mr. X on June 9, 2013?"

(A) "Yes."
(B) "I think I was there."
(C) "If I was scheduled that day, I took care of him."
(D) "I may have."

Answers

A-401

(A), (C), and (E) Fever occurs in most clients in the presence of infection but may not occur in older adults, immunocompromised clients, clients who have malnutrition or those who have chronic alcohol or drug abuse, clients who have kidney or liver failure, and clients receiving corticosteroids or immunotherapy. A client who is receiving chemotherapy is often immunocompromised.

A-402

(A) When giving testimony the nurse should just say "yes" or "no" whenever possible without adding detail. In this case, the nurse should just confirm that care was given that day and give no further information.

Q–403

The nurse is caring for a client and wants to ensure that the client understands all of the aspects of the Patient Self-Determination Act. What information will the nurse share with this client? Select all that apply.

(A) HIPPA privacy rights
(B) Living will
(C) Durable power of attorney for health care
(D) Patient Care Partnership
(E) Do not resuscitate orders

Q–404

A graduate nurse is concerned about action taken against the nurse's license. Which persons may notify the state board of nursing of a breach of law by the nurse?

(A) The healthcare facility that employs that nurse
(B) The nurse's direct supervisor
(C) Only the individual who observed the alleged breach of law
(D) Any individual who wishes to bring a charge against the nurse's license

Answers

A–403

(B), **(C)**, and **(E)** The Patient Self-Determination Act involves advance directives (living will and durable power of attorney for health care) and DNR orders written by a healthcare provider. The HIPPA privacy rights and the Patient Care Partnership are a part of client rights.

A–404

(D) Any person may contact the state board of nursing and bring a charge against an individual nurse. It may be brought by an individual and by the employer, but it also may come from a client or a client's family member or an acquaintance of the nurse.

Safe and Effective Care Environment:
Coordinated Care

Q-405

Which of the following situations could be considered HIPPA violations? Select all that apply.

(A) The nurse throws a paper with client information in the trash at the end of the shift.
(B) The nurse logs off the computer after charting.
(C) The nurse discusses a client incident with another nurse in a locked conference room.
(D) The nurse talks to the client about the results of a diagnostic test with visitors present in the client's room.
(E) The nurse leaves a voice message for an obstetrical client about upcoming prenatal appointments.

Safe and Effective Care Environment:
Safety and Infection Control

Q-406

The nurse is caring for a client who has been admitted to the oncology unit for treatment with internal radiation. What nursing action is most important for the nurse to remember when caring for this client?

(A) Teach the client where to dispose of his urine and feces while the internal radiation is in place.
(B) Organize nursing care activities to limit the amount of time with the client.
(C) Use the time with the client to assist with comfort measures such as a back massage.
(D) Wear gloves and a surgical mask while in the client's room.

Answers

A–405

(A), (D), and (E) At the end of the shift, the nurse must discard all client notes in a secure place that could not be accessed by unauthorized persons. Medical information should only be discussed with the client in private. The nurse must first obtain permission before proceeding with a conversation about the client's test results. Messages that identify a client's condition (such as pregnancy) should not be left on a voicemail without client permission.

A–406

(B) It is important that the nurse organize nursing care activities that limit time with the client to limit the amount of radiation a nurse will receive while in the client's room. The client is discouraged from moving around to prevent the internal radiation from becoming dislodged. The nurse should not only limit time in the client's room but also limit the time the nurse is in close proximity to the client, so activities such as back rubs should be avoided. The nurse should wear protective shielding such as a lead apron and a film badge to monitor the amount of radiation the nurse receives. Gloves and a surgical mask will not provide protection to the nurse.

Questions

Safe and Effective Care Environment:
Safety and Infection Control

Q–407

The nurse is leading a group discussion about poisoning and knows that which substance is the leading cause of poisoning in the United States?

(A) Lead poisoning
(B) Prescription drugs
(C) Household chemicals
(D) House plants

Safe and Effective Care Environment:
Safety and Infection Control

Q–408

The nurse is caring for a client who suddenly begins to vomit and the nurse's face is splashed with vomitus. What is the first step the nurse should take in this situation?

(A) Call the nursing supervisor.
(B) Inform the infection control nurse.
(C) Wash the face with liberal amounts of water.
(D) Wipe the vomitus off the face with a paper towel.

| 413

A–407

(B) Most poisoning occurs because of the misuse or abuse of prescription drugs. All other substances can cause poisoning especially among children but the greatest increase in poisonings is among adults and is related to abuse of opioid analgesics.

A–408

(C) In the event of an unexpected exposure to possible blood-borne pathogens, the nurse should minimize the exposure by washing the area thoroughly. Then the nurse should notify the appropriate personnel and fill out the necessary paperwork.

Q–409

The nurse is preparing to perform a surgical scrub prior to entering a neonatal intensive care unit. What step is most important for the nurse to perform prior to beginning the surgical scrub?

(A) Wash hands with soap and water.
(B) Clean under the fingernails.
(C) Put a surgical mask on.
(D) Put on sterile shoes.

Q–410

The home health nurse is caring for a client with a small wound that is infected with MRSA. What instructions are most important for the nurse to share with this client to prevent spread of the infection to other members of the family?

(A) Use plasticware for meals and immediately dispose of it in a separate trash can.
(B) Use a cotton handkerchief to cover a sneeze or cough.
(C) Leave the infected area open to air but covered with antibiotic ointment.
(D) Shower daily with antibacterial soap.

A–409

(A) Before proceeding with a surgical scrub, the nurse must first wash the hands with soap and water. Cleaning under the finger-nails will occur with the surgical scrub. The nurse will put on the surgical attire before beginning the hand washing and surgical scrub.

A–410

(D) Clients who have MRSA do not have to use plasticware for meals but should avoid sharing personal items such as towels, makeup, combs, and clothing. The client should use paper tissues and cough and sneeze into the elbow. The wound that is infected with MRSA should always be covered with a bandage. The client should wear gloves when changing the dressing. The client should shower daily using antibacterial soap.

Safe and Effective Care Environment:
Safety and Infection Control

Q–411

The nurse is caring for a client who is in isolation due to an infection that is transmitted by droplet. The nurse will assist the client in dealing with the effects of isolation in what ways? Select all that apply.

(A) Inform the client that only healthcare facility employees must wear protective equipment.

(B) Occasionally open the client's door and talk to the client without a mask.

(C) Remove gloves when preparing to touch the client.

(D) Spend time talking to the client about the isolation.

(E) Let the client know that the isolation measures will be removed as soon as possible.

Safe and Effective Care Environment:
Coordinated Care

Q–412

The nurse is caring for a client who is alert and oriented but has been recently diagnosed with a terminal illness. The client's companion says to the nurse, "I will be making all of the healthcare decisions for my friend because I have been designated his durable power of attorney (DPOA) for health care." What is the nurse's best response?

(A) "That's good to know. I will review the healthcare provider's orders with you."

(B) "That may only be used if your friend is unable to make his own decisions."

(C) "You will then need to stay at your friend's bedside around the clock in case you are needed."

(D) "Do you have your friend's living will that documents this?"

A–411

(B), **(D)**, and **(E)** It may be difficult for clients to cope with isolation. It is important for the nurse to let the client know that it is temporary. The nurse should spend time talking with the client while giving care and because droplet infection is only contagious at three feet, the nurse can occasionally open the client's door and talk to the client without a mask. The nurse should touch the client while in the room but always wear gloves and anyone coming into the client's room, including family, must wear the appropriate protective equipment.

A–412

(B) A durable power of attorney (DPOA) for health care is used when an individual indicates another individual to make healthcare decisions if the first individual is unable to do so. That is the only time it is to be used. Therefore, the nurse would not review the healthcare provider's orders with the friend because the client is alert and oriented. It is not necessary for the individual with the DPOA to stay at the bedside, and the living will is a notarized document that lists the client's wishes in situations such as end-of-life care. It would not include the DPOA documentation.

Q–413

The LPN/LVN will be caring for four clients this shift. Which client should the LPN/LVN visit first?

(A) A 77-year-old client recovering from hip replacement surgery who has an oral temperature of 99.9° F.
(B) A 62-year-old client with left hemiparesis who needs to use the bathroom.
(C) A 72-year-old client who had a left lower leg amputation and is complaining of severe indigestion.
(D) A 90-year-old client with COPD who is confused and asking for his mother.

Q–414

The nurse is caring for a client admitted with a urinary tract infection. The client experienced a fall while attempting to get out of bed without assistance. Which is the best documentation of the event?

(A) Client found on floor, 2 cm laceration to forehead, client alert, B/P 117/80, P-94, R-16.
(B) Client fell on floor attempting to get out of bed. Small cut on head. Bandage applied.
(C) Client tried to get out of bed and fell. Adhesive bandage applied to head.
(D) Healthcare provider notified that client experienced a fall while getting out of bed.

A–413

(C) Any client who complaints of chest pain (severe indigestion) must be assessed before anyone else.

A–414

(A) The most complete documentation is the one that describes the client's condition and doesn't editorialize. In this case, the nurse documents where the client was found, what was found, and what the client's vital signs were. It does not include what the nurse thinks might have happened (for example, fell out of bed) or any generalizations about the client.

Safe and Effective Care Environment:
Coordinated Care

Q–415

Which statement by the nurse demonstrates the ethical value of veracity?

(A) "I'll be back with your medication in five minutes."
(B) "The medication that I administered was not the right dosage."
(C) "I will support you in whatever decision you make."
(D) "I am only able to spend the next five minutes talking to you."

Psychosocial Integrity

Q–416

The nurse is caring for a 15-year-old female who has been admitted with electrolyte imbalances related to anorexia nervosa. Which nursing intervention will best promote weight gain in this client?

(A) Weigh the client daily at the same time every day.
(B) Keep a strict record of intake and output.
(C) Stay with the client during meals and for an hour after meals.
(D) Discuss each food that the client is eating and the number of calories eaten.

A–415

(B) Veracity is the duty to tell the truth. The nurse demonstrates this value by informing the client that the wrong dosage of medication was administered. The nurse demonstrates fidelity (faithfulness) by returning to see the client as promised. The nurse demonstrates autonomy by supporting the client's decision, and the nurse demonstrates justice by explaining that there is limited time available to see the client and still take care of other clients.

A–416

(C) The best nursing intervention to promote weight gain in a client with anorexia nervosa is to stay with a client during established times for meals and for at least one hour following meals. Weighing the client and recording intake and output monitors the client's weight and electrolyte status but does not promote weight gain. The nurse should refrain from focusing the discussion on food and eating because these are not the real issues and would not promote weight gain.

Psychosocial Integrity

Q–417

The nurse is talking with a client who has come to the clinic because of a rapid heartbeat. The client is having great difficulty listening to the nurse's questions and is unable to complete the clinic intake paperwork. The nurse believes that the client's symptoms may be related to what type of psychological response?

(A) Mild anxiety
(B) Moderate anxiety
(C) Severe anxiety
(D) Panic anxiety

Psychosocial Integrity

Q–418

The nurse is caring for a young child who sustained a facial injury and notices that the mother is hesitant to pick up and cuddle the child when he cries. What would be the best response by the nurse to this situation?

(A) "I know your child looks different now but you will get used to it."
(B) "You need to pick up your child. He will think you don't love him."
(C) "Just close your eyes when you pick up your child and pretty soon it will be all right."
(D) "Can you share with me what you are feeling right now?"

Answers

A–417

(C) Severe anxiety manifests itself with physical symptoms such as headaches, palpitations, and insomnia and with emotional symptoms such as confusion, dread, and horror. The client has a very limited attention span and has great difficulty completing simple tasks. The client with panic-level anxiety may experience hallucinations or delusions and become extremely withdrawn. The client at this level of anxiety is unable to focus on even one detail within the environment. Clients with moderate anxiety are less able to concentrate but do not have the physical symptoms. A client with mild anxiety has a sharpened sense of the environment and learning is enhanced.

A–418

(D) It is important for the nurse to give this mother the opportunity to discuss what issue is disturbing her. The nurse can't assume the mother is hesitant to pick up the child because of the facial injury. The nurse also should not give the mother advice or shame the mother.

Q-419

The nurse is caring for a client who has lost the ability to speak. What is the best interpretation of a grimace on the client's face?

(A) The client is frustrated.
(B) The client is in pain.
(C) The client is surprised.
(D) The client is disinterested.

Psychosocial Integrity

Q-420

The nurse is caring for a client who has just been admitted to the unit with cirrhosis of the liver caused by chronic alcohol intake. What aspect of the client's history is most important for the nurse to assess in this client?

(A) "How long ago was your last alcoholic drink?"
(B) "When were you first diagnosed with cirrhosis?"
(C) "When did you first begin drinking?"
(D) "Do you attend Alcoholics Anonymous meetings?"

Answers

A–419

(B) Facial expressions can communicate a lot of information when the client is unable to speak. A grimace indicates fear or pain. Compressed lips indicate frustration. Widening of the eyes indicates surprise or enthusiasm. A stare indicates dislike or disinterest.

A–420

(A) It is most important for the nurse to assess when the client had his last drink to assess when the possible symptoms of alcohol withdrawal would begin. The other questions would provide information to the nurse but are not important at this time.

Q–421

The nurse is caring for four clients. Which client is most likely to receive the services of a nurse case manager?

(A) An 8-year-old client who had an emergency appendectomy
(B) A 23-year-old client with type 1 diabetes mellitus and renal failure
(C) A 44-year-old client with community-acquired pneumonia
(D) A 67-year-old client who had a bilateral oophorectomy

Q–422

Which of the following actions will be the best at containing healthcare costs for a client?

(A) Ensure that all client documentation is complete.
(B) Ambulate the client frequently to make sure that client is ready for discharge.
(C) Reuse dressing supplies when providing wound care.
(D) Complete client care as quickly as possible to ensure efficiency.

Answers

A–421

(B) A case manager is often responsible for a specific group of clients. It is usually those clients who are the sickest, experience chronic illness, or experience complications. The client with both diabetes and renal failure would be the most likely client to received case management services. The other clients have a greater chance of having a short-term hospitalization with little chance of complications.

A–422

(A) The most important thing that the LPN/LVN can do in containing healthcare costs is to make certain that client documentation is complete and includes all supplies used and all procedures completed. This ensures that the healthcare facility receives all of the reimbursement that it deserves for the care given to this client. It is important to ambulate the client, but it is not the most important aspect of cost containment. Supplies should be reused if possible, but supplies for wound care should not be reused because they may contaminate the wound. Client care should be completed as efficiently as possible but efficient does not mean fast. Client care that is given too quickly may mean that the early signs of a complication may be missed.

Safe and Effective Care Environment:
Coordinated Care

Q–423

The nurse is caring for a client who has a spinal cord injury that has resulted in paralysis from the waist down. During morning assessment, the client's blood pressure is 210/150 and the client is complaining of a severe headache. What is the nurse's first action in the care of this client?

(A) Request the charge nurse to retake the blood pressure.
(B) Obtain the ordered prn medication for headache.
(C) Raise the head of the client's bed.
(D) Place 2 L of oxygen by nasal cannula on the client.

Safe and Effective Care Environment:
Coordinated Care

Q–424

The nurse is caring for four clients who all require medications at 0800. Which client will the nurse medicate first?

(A) The client with myasthenia gravis who has neostigmine ordered.
(B) The client who had a colectomy and has requested hydromorphone who rates pain at a 9 out of 10.
(C) The client with pneumonia who requires acetaminophen for an oral temperature of 103.4° F.
(D) The client with a seizure disorder who receives a daily dose of phenytoin.

A–423

(C) The client with a spinal cord injury who develops hypertension and a severe headache is showing symptoms of autonomic dysreflexia, which is an emergency situation. The nurse should raise the head of the client's bed to relieve the precipitating problem. For clients with this condition, it is often caused by a full bladder or impacted stool. The nurse does not need to wait to have someone else take the blood pressure. The medication that may be given would be for reduction of blood pressure, not medication for the headache. Placing oxygen on the client would not relieve the problem.

A–424

(A) The client with myasthenia gravis must be the first client to receive medication because the client must have a continuous level of medication to be able to swallow and ultimately to breathe. The other clients have a need to be medicated as soon as possible, but they must wait until the client with myasthenia gravis receives the medication that ensures the ability to swallow.

Safe and Effective Care Environment:
Coordinated Care

Q–425

A client has been receiving an opioid analgesic prn every four hours for treatment of pain related to a femur fracture. What is the most important nursing intervention the nurse should perform when the client requests pain medication four hours after the last administration of pain medication?

(A) Document the client's current pain rating.
(B) Assess the client's respirations.
(C) Encourage the client to use distraction for pain control.
(D) Administer the pain medication.

Answers

A–425

(B) Opioid medications can cause respiratory depression so the most important action by the nurse when the client requests a pain medication after ensuring it is time to give it is to assess the client's respirations. The client would not be able to receive an opioid analgesic if the respirations were at 10 or below. Then the nurse can assess the client's pain rating and administer the pain medication. The nurse can also suggest possible distractions that may assist a client who is experiencing pain.

Index

Index

Index

Index